Get Your Lower Back Pain under Control –

and Get on with Life

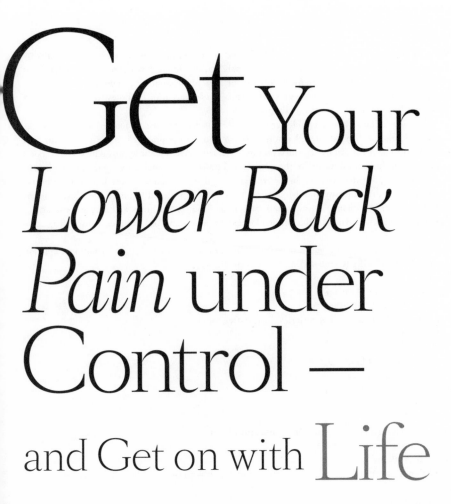

Get Your *Lower Back Pain* under Control —

and Get on with Life

Anthony H. Guarino, M.D.

The Johns Hopkins University Press
Baltimore

Note to the reader: Diet, exercise programs, and the use of medications are all matters that by their very nature vary from individual to individual. You should speak with your own doctor about your individual needs before beginning any diet or exercise program. It is especially important to discuss the use of any medications with your doctor. These precautionary notes are most important if you are already under medical care for an illness.

Drug dosage: The author and publisher have made reasonable efforts to determine that the selection and dosage of drugs discussed in this text conform to the practices of the general medical community. The medications described do not necessarily have specific approval by the U.S. Food and Drug Administration for use in the diseases and dosages for which they are recommended. In view of ongoing research, changes in governmental regulations, and the constant flow of information relating to drug therapy and drug reactions, the reader is urged to check the package insert of each drug for any change in indications and dosage and for warnings and precautions. This is particularly important when the recommended agent is a new and/or infrequently used drug.

The author is a speaker and educator for several pharmaceutical companies, including Cephalon (Amrix, Fentora), Lilly (Cymbalta), and Wyeth (Relistor).

© 2010 Anthony H. Guarino
All rights reserved. Published 2010
Printed in the United States of America on acid-free paper
9 8 7 6 5 4 3 2 1

The Johns Hopkins University Press
2715 North Charles Street
Baltimore, Maryland 21218-4363
www.press.jhu.edu

Library of Congress Cataloging-in-Publication Data

Guarino, Anthony H.
    Get your lower back pain under control—and get on with life / Anthony H. Guarino.
        p. cm.
    Includes index.
    ISBN-13: 978-0-8018-9730-6 (hardcover : alk. paper)
    ISBN-10: 0-8018-9730-0 (hardcover : alk. paper)
    ISBN-13: 978-0-8018-9731-3 (pbk. : alk. paper)
    ISBN-10: 0-8018-9731-9 (pbk. : alk. paper)
    1. Backache—Popular works. I. Title.
RD771.B217G83 2010
617.5'64—dc22   2010001249

A catalog record for this book is available from the British Library.

Illustrations on pages 165, 166, 168, 169, 171, and 173 by Jacqueline Schaffer.

Special discounts are available for bulk purchases of this book. For more information, please contact Special Sales at 410-516-6936 or specialsales@press.jhu.edu.

The Johns Hopkins University Press uses environmentally friendly book materials, including recycled text paper that is composed of at least 30 percent post-consumer waste, whenever possible. All of our book papers are acid-free, and our jackets and covers are printed on paper with recycled content.

Contents

Part III. The Cost of Chronic Pain

Preface

My greatest insights into the nature of low back pain come from my patients.

YOU KNOW IT IF you have it—a constant pain low in your back that never leaves. It's always there. You seek out new doctors. You try new medications. You participate in a specialized exercise regimen. You even try to work on your attitude, because you've heard that if you can alter your perception of pain, you can alter the pain itself.

Some days are good days, and you are hopeful. Other days are particularly painful, and you try not to despair. You view the world through the distorted lens of your ever-present pain. You wonder if you will ever get any relief.

As director of pain management services at Barnes-Jewish West County Hospital and as faculty at Washington University School of Medicine, I help people with all kinds of pain—and all the problems that go along with having lots of pain or having pain that lasts a long time. The sheer number of my patients who experience low back pain has inspired me to focus my attention on those who suffer from this devastating condition and to find a way to make a difference in their lives. My patients have shown me how low back pain alters their lives—and their family's lives, too. Low back pain can cause or worsen depression and addiction, can cause or contribute to disability and divorce. Individuals suffer, families suffer, and ultimately society as a whole suffers.

I wrote this book to offer hope and guidance for anyone affected by low back pain. In this book you will discover that managing pain means taking a multipronged approach. You can become stronger, and regain confidence and peace in your life, by learning what causes pain and then actively participating with your doctor and other therapists to treat and manage your pain.

Over years of treating people, I have come to understand that the psychological benefits of pain management are as important as the physical ones. Pain's reach goes way beyond sensation. It invades emotions and interferes with relationships. It skews a person's view of him- or herself and the surrounding world. It can rob people of spirituality and cause them to doubt their beliefs. But just as an injured soldier must practice walking, talking, and any number of other functions that he or she used to take for granted, people who suffer from chronic back pain must persevere. If *you* suffer with chronic back pain, you must work with determination and self-control to modify your pain state and take back control of your body. Even with these efforts you may not be pain free, but you will be able to function better at home and in the workplace, and find enjoyment in life.

Back pain is the most common cause of chronic pain in the United States. By some estimates, it affects 80 percent of adults at some time during their life.[1] While you don't wish suffering on others, there is something consoling in knowing you are not alone.

Anyone with back pain is going to do better if he or she understands the nature of pain—the anatomical components and emotional components of it. Part 1 of this book explains pain and also offers guidance for choosing a doctor and what to expect when you visit a doctor, including how a diagnosis is made and why a specific therapy is recommended. Readers who want more detail should consult the detailed anatomical descriptions and illustrations in the appendix. Part 2 of the book describes the full range of medical interventions to be had, from physical therapy and exercise to injections, medications, and surgery. If you are aware of all the options available to help you with your pain, you will be much better equipped to ask informed questions of your doctor and work with your doctor to get you feeling better.

Because the cost of chronic pain can be high, both in dollars and in time lost from work, insurance and disability coverage are often a concern for people with low back pain. In part 3, I turn to these topics, and

I discuss relationships, as well. Even the strongest of relationships can be tested when chronic pain interferes with daily life. Some of the people who care about you may not understand what you are going through, and you may not fully understand how your pain is affecting their lives. Chapter 13 will guide you to use your relationships as an incentive to take back control of your life.

My patients have taught me many lessons that can't be found in medical books. I hope everyone reading this book will benefit from what my patients *and* my medical books have taught me. Feel better, and get back into life.

Part I

Why Does It Hurt?
Who Can Help?

Chapter 1
All about Pain

After head colds, low back pain is the most common reason to visit a physician.

LOW BACK PAIN IS one of the most common conditions in the United States, affecting approximately 80 percent of the adult population at some time in their lives.[1] Back pain affects men and women of all races. The highest incidence of low back pain reported to doctors is among people 35 to 55 years old.

The prevalence of this condition has enormous financial and socioeconomic implications:

- Low back pain is one of the most commonly given reasons for absence from work in this country—second only to coughs and colds.
- About half of the people who are employed in the United States have back problems every year—that's one out of every two working Americans.
- Low back pain is cited as the most frequent complaint in workers' compensation claims and the most common reason for early Social Security disability payouts. The total medical cost to treat back pain exceeds $80 billion annually.
- Back pain is the most common reason why individuals under the age of 55 limit activity, the fifth most common reason for admission to the hospital, and the third ranking reason for surgical intervention.

- Research has shown that approximately 1 percent of the population in the United States is considered permanently disabled from back conditions, with an additional 1 percent temporarily disabled from back conditions.[2]

The Physiology of Pain | The many ways that pain affects us

The International Association for the Study of Pain defines the mechanism of pain as an "unpleasant sensory and emotional experience associated with actual or potential tissue damage" (www.iasp-pain.org). The society recognizes that if you suffer from pain, you feel it, it is not pleasant, it may affect your emotions, and you may experience real tissue damage now or in the future. The way pain affects you can, in fact, be divided into six different categories: biological, psychological, behavioral, cognitive, spiritual, and cultural.

The *biological* effect is what most people associate with the word "pain." It is a signal to the body that an injury has occurred. Think about the last time you attempted to remove a hot cup from the microwave. That burning sensation in your hand as you quickly put down the cup is an example of the biological manifestation of pain. Similarly, the lower back sends a message to your brain that there is a problem, alerting you to change how you move to avoid increasing the damage.

Studies have more recently documented the *psychological,* or emotional, effects of pain. Constant suffering can cause depression, anxiety, and insomnia, which are potentially life-altering or even life-threatening conditions.

The *behavioral* effects of pain change how a person moves or acts. If you twist your ankle while walking down the street, the resulting pain will cause you to alter the way you walk, and you may limp to compensate for the injury. For people with chronic back pain that compensation may mean using a cane, walking hunched over, or leaning to one side. When you suffer from pain, you will try to minimize that pain by experimenting with different physical positions, diet and exercise as appropriate, medications, and possibly surgery, if needed.

Pain impacts us *cognitively* by forcing us to think about it in an effort to determine what's causing it and what we can do to get rid of it. Perhaps this is why you are reading this book right now.

Pain affects us *spiritually* by reminding us that we are, in fact, human and, as such, vulnerable and mortal. Pain leads us to question its purpose and our own role in that larger picture. It helps us to change what we can and accept what we cannot change.

The *cultural* effects of pain are the lifestyle changes that occur in avoidance of pain, like using a treadmill instead of running on the pavement, avoiding long car trips, or eliminating activities that may involve heavy lifting. Pain is a complex process that touches many aspects of our lives.

Acute Pain versus Chronic Pain | What is the difference?

Acute pain is triggered by tissue damage resulting from illness, injury, or surgery. It is self-limiting, which means it doesn't last longer than a few weeks or months. The word *acute* comes from the Latin word "needle," referring to a sharp pain. Touching a hot pan causes acute pain. The source of the pain is the pan, which stimulates the pain receptors in the hand and causes us to withdraw the hand from the pan. You can pinpoint the area where the burn and the pain occurred. Once the burn heals, you will no longer have pain. People suffering from chronic pain have no such reassurance.

Chronic pain occurs long after an injury has healed. Medically, we consider pain chronic if it lasts longer than six months. The word *chronic* comes from the Greek word for "time." Like acute pain, it can be described as tingling, jolting, burning, dull, sharp, or throbbing. It can be continuous or it can come and go.

The cause of chronic pain is unclear and therefore not well understood. Often, there is no evidence of disease or damage to the body that a doctor can easily link to the pain. Examples of chronic pain states can include back pain, fibromyalgia, diabetic neuropathy, and headaches. A slight variation is a form of pain that is both chronic and intermittent, in that it comes and goes. Examples of "chronic intermittent pain" include migraines, irritable bowel syndrome, and rheumatoid arthritis.

The Role of the Nervous System | How messages are sent

The nervous system plays a starring role in the sensation of pain. Two types of nerve fibers relay messages to our spinal cord and brain: A–delta fibers and C fibers. The A–delta fibers respond first and the C fibers, considered peripheral nerves, respond second.

Under normal circumstances, A–delta fibers serve as a warning system. The nerves respond to the damaging extremes of heat or cold, accidental or surgical trauma, and inflammation. As a rule, sensory nerves bring information to the spinal cord regarding pain and other sensations, such as heat, cold, vibration, or touch. The spinal cord takes the information, modifies it, and then distributes it to the nerves, which are in turn responsible for relaying the information to the brain.

Some circumstances, however, activate another set of nerves. The best example of how this second set, or C fibers, works, is to think about what happens when you hit your funny bone, the ulnar nerve in your arm. The first sensation you feel is a sharp, tingling pain. This is a result of A–delta fiber activity. Your early warning nerves carry the message that you just hit your funny bone directly to the spinal cord at approximately 40 miles per hour. The second sensation you feel is an aching that slowly spreads up and down the inner side of your arm. This aching is caused by the C fibers, which carry their message at a rate of 3 miles per hour to the spinal cord. The difference in the rate of speed explains the difference in pain perception.

The Role of the Spinal Cord | The body's gatekeeper

Think of the sensory nerves as a highway and the spinal cord as the tollbooth that allows for messages sent by the nerves to be modified, re-sent, or canceled prior to traveling on to the brain. This concept is known as the *gate theory* and it aptly describes one of the important functions of our spinal cord.

Specific areas of the spinal cord are responsible for magnifying the pain message in order to allow for a release of amino acids known as Substance P. Substance P expands the area of receptivity to incoming pain signals. Medical science has not yet determined why this occurs, but it does.

When a pain signal travels to the brain, the brain interprets whether it is a normal or an abnormal message. The brain can alter the message by releasing impulses that reconfigure the message or by releasing endorphins, which decrease the intensity of the signal. The brain gives meaning to the pain message, which is why we grimace, limp, or cry in response to the signal. However, when the brain and the spinal cord are bombarded with a high level of intense pain signals, they eventually lose the ability to provide these normal checks and balances. This is what can happen to a person who suffers from chronic pain.

The Role of Inflammation | When it works and when it hurts

Inflammation is a process designed to fight infection or repair tissue damage caused by an injury. When it is working properly, it plays a vital role in our body's response system; when it is out of control, chronic pain can result.

Think about the last time you fell and scraped your knee. After sustaining the fall, you experienced a quick succession of events: the cells in the damaged area released chemicals that irritated the pain nerves, causing those nerves to send out a signal to the spinal cord, which in turn made you aware that an injury had occurred. At the same time, muscle spasms developed to further protect the area by restricting movement. Blood vessels in the surrounding area constricted to reduce bleeding from the site. Lastly, white blood cells and other connective tissue cells started the cleanup process. In chronic pain states, such as rheumatoid arthritis, an inflammatory process may be out of control; instead of repairing any damage, it makes the natural health of tissues worse. In this disease state, it is thought that the body is attacking itself. Symptoms can wax and wane and corresponding destructive changes to synovial joints may occur.

Neuropathic Pain | When the nervous system malfunctions

Neuropathic pain is a state caused by an injury or a dysfunction in the nervous system, such as an infection. Injury to the nervous system that results in chronic pain can occur anywhere from the peripheral nerve terminal in the skin to the cerebral cortex in the skull. Neuropathic pain is distinguished from other types in that the sensory symptoms persist beyond the typical healing period.

Examples of neuropathic pain syndrome include phantom (stump) pain following an amputation; diabetic neuropathy, where the blood flow is altered causing numbness, tingling, or pain; and postherpetic neuralgia experienced by many people who develop shingles, where a virus that has remained dormant after a childhood bout with chickenpox manifests itself later in life through the nerves causing itching, rashes, and persistent pain.

One of the most common disease states associated with neuropathic pain is diabetes. Other examples are hypothyroidism, alcoholism, AIDS, and multiple myeloma. The symptoms most often associated with neuropathic pain include spontaneous burning, shooting pain, numbness or tingling of the affected area, and a condition called allodynia, in which the sensation of pain results from a stimulus that would not usually cause pain, such as a light touch of the skin.

In neuropathic pain, the central nervous system—the combination of the brain and spinal cord—undergoes changes with the peripheral nerve injury. The good news is that research has shown that pain messages can be interrupted. Technically stated, stimulation and propagation of the large fiber (A-beta) sensory inputs could override painful neuropathic sensory inputs, thus reducing the perceived intensity of pain. This mechanism is what happens when we shake or rub an injured body part and thereby reduce our pain perception.

How can this information help you? Well, have you ever noticed that if you hit your finger with a hammer, your back doesn't hurt as much as it did? Pain signals go through a gate before being sent to the brain, and "the squeaky wheel gets the grease." (In this case, the squeaky wheel is the overwhelmingly urgent pain from the finger.) Similarly, medical and other treatments can control or alter the messages and pain signals that are going through the gate in an effort to cause the spinal cord to reach an imbalanced state. This imbalanced state confuses the painful and nonpainful impulses in a way that affects the signals that are going to the brain.

Causes of Low Back Pain | Why is this happening?

Low back pain is caused by several different factors, including problems with muscles, ligaments, or nerves, disc problems, or stress. Muscles or ligaments that have been injured or irritated, such as with a strain, can cause pain. Did you exercise too vigorously? Did you lift something too heavy? Did you twist your body in a quick movement? If you have low back pain that coincides with pain radiating down one or both legs, you may have a disc problem. The disc is a cushion that sits between the bones of your spine. Over time and with activity the cushion can bulge or *herniate* out of its usual space. This bulging can press on the nerves, causing an irritation that in turn causes pain to travel down the leg. *(Note: The anatomy of the back and many of the technical terms used in this chapter are described and illustrated in the appendix.)*

Another reason for back pain is stress. The pain may start, continue, or worsen during an emotionally stressful time. Stress, whether conscious or unconscious, causes the muscles in the back to tighten, which results in pain.

Description of Low Back Pain | Its symptoms

Think about whether you suffer from one or more of the following characteristics of low back pain:

- Have you felt a throbbing, aching, shooting, stabbing, or dull quality pain in your back?
- Does the pain go up or down or radiate to one or both legs, with little or no pain in your back?
- Do you have a feeling of numbness or weakness in one or both legs?
- Do problems with your sleep result in decreased energy or feelings of depression or anxiety?
- Does your pain move to different parts of the body, including the back or arms?
- Do you have pain that is made worse by stress or emotional issues?

These are just a few of the typical symptoms that accompany low back pain. If you answered yes to one or more of these questions, you may indeed suffer from low back pain.

A Range of Practitioners | Who can help?

A variety of health care providers can treat low back pain utilizing a wide range of traditional and nontraditional methods. In looking for treatment, most patients start with their general practitioner. Primary care physicians have general training in all areas of medicine and can determine whether more specialized care is needed; they may refer you to an anesthesiologist, a chiropractor, a neurologist, a neurosurgeon, an orthopedist, an osteopath, or a physiatrist. Be aware that back pain often resolves on its own, with little or no treatment. Let's look at each of these specialists in alphabetical order and see how they might help you.

An *anesthesiologist* has specialized training in treating pain problems because this area of medicine focuses on decreasing a person's perception of pain. The treatment approach could include medication management, spinal injections, or physical therapy.

A *chiropractor* restores normal function of the spine through a series of manipulations. Chiropractic is based on the belief that misaligned vertebrae restrict the spine's ability to move and ultimately affect the nerves that radiate from the spine, and that abnormal function in the nervous system causes disease states to occur. Chiropractors utilize massage therapy, physical therapy, nutritional counseling, and vitamin therapy in their practice. They aim to realign the vertebrae, restore range of motion, and improve the nerve pathways. Spinal manipulation can be effective for uncomplicated low back pain, especially if the pain has been present for less than a month.

The most common form of chiropractic treatment for low back pain is spinal manipulation therapy, in which the practitioner utilizes joint manipulation of the spine and extremities (arms and legs). Chiropractors also use stretching and modalities such as heat and cold applications. Several sessions may be required before the patient notices an improvement in pain level. Chiropractors must be extremely careful in manipulating the neck; some spinal cord injuries have occurred during manipulation, though rarely.

Neurologists are medical doctors who specialize in the nervous system. They use nonsurgical techniques and treatment to diagnose and treat back pain. *Neurosurgeons*, on the other hand, focus on the surgical treatment of nervous system problems.

Orthopedists, also medical doctors, specialize in the surgical treatment of skeletal problems. Common orthopedic surgeries include knee and hip replacements, joint surgery, and spinal surgery, such as a laminectomy or discectomy.

An *osteopath* is a doctor of osteopathy (D.O.) who practices similarly to a medical doctor (M.D.) but who may also incorporate conventional medical, surgical, and pharmacological principles with chiropractic techniques such as manipulation of the spine to address general musculo-skeletal problems.

Finally, a *physiatrist*, not to be confused with a psychiatrist, is a medical doctor who focuses on patient rehabilitation, especially after stroke or injury to a muscle or joint.

Most of these specialties will be discussed in greater detail in the next chapter. Let me state here ("for the record," as the saying goes) that I am an anesthesiologist. My aim is to help you the reader to understand pain and treatments for pain, and how you can reclaim your life with the knowledge this book imparts.

Emergencies | When to seek immediate help

Certain symptoms of back pain should not be ignored because they in fact signal that you have a medical emergency. If you suddenly lose control of your bowel or bladder you should be seen in the emergency room immediately. Bowel or bladder problems include difficulty in controlling or initiating the urine stream or bowel movement, no feeling in the groin or anal area, or the inability to achieve an erection. Any of these symptoms indicate the possibility of "cauda equina syndrome," a situation where the nerves that control the bowel and bladder become compressed or flat. If the situation is not corrected in 24 to 48 hours, the damage may be permanent.

Weakness in the legs or feet also constitutes an emergency, and you must seek medical attention immediately. If you experience a dragging of your foot, called foot drop, it may be the result of an inability to flex your foot and toes up toward your head—which would be a sign of weakness. Back pain that awakens you from sleep can indicate the presence of a tumor or spinal infection. This situation is called "rest pain" and can be described as severe throbbing and aching that is actually made worse by rest.

In general, if you are involved in a motor vehicle accident or sustain any type of fall, imaging studies should be done to rule out trauma to the spine. Or if back pain is so severe that it impairs function and ordinary daily activities, you should see a doctor immediately or be evaluated in the nearest emergency room.

If you do not have any of the above symptoms, it is less likely that you have a medical emergency and the best course in that case may be to let the pain be your guide. Using bed rest in short stints, taking anti-inflammatories, and rotating ice and heat is the best course of action. Use ice for 20 minutes every 4 hours for the first 24 hours, then switch to heat for 20 minutes every 4 hours for the next 24 hours. After 48 hours, there is no concrete rule for alternating ice and heat, though some people have a routine that they swear by.

If the pain persists, seek help from your doctor. Your doctor will perform a thorough evaluation and design a treatment plan compatible with your needs, including referral to a specialist if needed.

Risk Factors for Back Pain | Who gets it?

Identifying risk factors that predispose an individual to low back pain is a daunting task given the complicated nature of the disease. In general, there are three classifications of risk factors associated with low back pain: physical or biomechanical, personal, and psychosocial. Physical factors include occupations that require frequent bending and lifting, working with the back in an awkward position, postural stress to the back, and operating vibrating equipment. These factors explain the frequency of low back pain reported in occupations such as construction work, driving, and nursing.

Personal risk factors include lifestyle, gender, age, weight, genetics, and poor general health. Lifestyle might account for the difference in back pain between a person who sits in a chair most of the day and a person who is active; as we will see in chapter 5, toning your core muscles and maintaining your strength through activity can help you avoid back pain in the first place. Although I know of no studies that support a claim that gender by itself is a risk factor, men suffer back pain more frequently than women because men still fill a larger percentage of the physically demanding jobs out there. Age plays a role in back pain because as a person ages, the tissue in the back becomes less elastic and degenerates, leading to increased vulnerability to pain. Excess weight is also a risk factor because obesity places additional strain on the structures of the back. If one or more of your parents had back problems, the likelihood that you too will experience some difficulties increases. And finally, poor general health affects a person in many ways, including back pain.

Psychosocial factors contributing to back pain are those circum-stances in patients' lives that are both psychological and social in nature. Conditions such as work environment, marital status, and a prior history of back pain can play a role. Job satisfaction is one of the most significant factors that consistently affects the frequency of low back pain; research has shown a connection between a worker's perception of the physical and psychosocial environment at work and actual pain. Psychological factors, especially depression, are clearly associated with low back pain, although research has not shown clearly whether depression precedes the incidence or follows the onset of pain.

Back pain affects many people, has diverse causes, and is treated by a variety of practitioners using numerous modalities. This book will help you sort through the various causes and treatments to find your way to a healthier back. The next chapter takes a closer look at the specialists who treat people with back pain—and how they go about it.

Chapter 2
The Right Doctor for You

Look for a physician who is board certified in pain management and who has a reputation for caring.

IN AN IDEAL WORLD, patients would be able to pick any doctor and get all the care they think they need whenever they need it. This level of choice and access to care may be available to patients who have the financial means to pay for care out of their own pockets—through concierge medical practices, for example. But most people rely on insurance to cover their medical care, and if a doctor doesn't accept a particular insurance plan, then the patient can't receive the care of that physician. In the real world, then, many factors influence which doctor a patient can see.

Some people believe they need to see "the best" doctor. That phrase makes me cringe, because many of the doctors who become known as "the best" are merely those who actively promote themselves. What a patient should look for in a physician is competence and an interest in helping the patient. A doctor who has received certification from a medical board is considered to be competent by others in his or her specialty. Board certification indicates competence. Whether a doctor is interested in helping the patient will be obvious during consultations. A doctor may have a great reputation with lots of certificates, but if he or she is not invested in helping you, you may be wasting your time.

People with chronic low back pain should find a physician whose practice focuses on this medical problem. Many doctors, including most primary care doctors, don't want to treat low back pain. They're apprehensive about prescribing narcotics to help people with chronic pain because they may still believe some myths about these medications—that treating a patient with narcotics will make him or her an addict, for instance. Most primary care doctors are not sufficiently trained to manage chronic low back pain, although some don't realize or admit it. Other physicians are not trained to take care of, or are not interested in taking care of, "the whole person," which is a necessity for patients with chronic pain.

There are a few primary care physicians who pass judgment on patients with chronic low back pain. If they haven't experienced low back pain themselves, they may question whether the pain is truly as incapacitating as the patient reports. Physicians generally are caring people, but not all of them have been appropriately educated on the nature of pain. Some of the problems that often go along with pain, such as insomnia, anxiety, and depression, make treatment even more challenging.

In the final analysis, trust your instincts. You will know when you and your doctor are a good fit. You will know when you are making progress.

Specialties | Who's who

In the previous chapter I briefly described the various health care providers who can treat back pain. In this chapter I will say more about what these specialists offer.

Anesthesiologists specialize in procedures that alleviate pain. They are experts in injectable medications. Many are also trained in nerve-destructive procedures such as radiofrequency neuroablation, which suspends the transmission of nerves, as well as nerve-modulating procedures, such as spinal cord stimulation. They are educated in the use of medications to alleviate pain. Many focus on injections as the only means to offer pain relief, which, as we will see, can be a disadvantage to the patient.

Neurologists have specialized training in understanding and treating problems in the nervous system. Some have received extra training in doing injections, and most are experts in using medications to alleviate pain. Even though they know much about medications, some still fear opioids, in spite of the fact that medical guidelines in their society (the American Academy of Neurology) clearly state that opioids are a first-line therapy for the treatment of neuropathic pain.

Physiatrists (Physical Medicine and Rehabilitation, or PMR) specialize in helping people restore function. Many are also trained in performing injections. They are more in tune with musculoskeletal problems than most specialists. Most physiatrists know about using medications, but some of them are not very aggressive about using pharmaceuticals in treatment. The organization for physiatrists is the American Academy of Physical Medicine and Rehabilitation.

Primary care doctors, such as family practitioners and internists, generally are not trained in the complete range of options available for effective treatment of low back pain. Instead, they most often have a general overall knowledge of all areas of medicine. Some do have an interest in managing pain and get the necessary instruction; and some obtain additional training in basic injections.

Psychiatrists specialize in treating psychological disease states with pharmaceuticals. A subset of this group may also focus on the treatment of chronic pain, and they prescribe narcotics to help manage pain. I would not expect a psychiatrist to know how to perform nerve-blocking injections (described in chapter 8). Most spend time listening to and counseling patients.

Pain Management Centers | Everything you need under one roof

Most people have their pain managed by physicians in individual practices. In the best-case scenario, these doctors are familiar with the various other disciplines necessary to treat pain. An alternative to the individual practice approach is a pain management center where all the disciplines necessary to manage pain exist under one roof; they may incorporate the expertise of all the specialties involved in managing pain, including anesthesia, physiatry, psychiatry, neurology, and surgery. Supporting their efforts will be a staff of well-trained nurses who do most of the patient education in the office.

Depending upon the size of the center, other specialists may also be on the staff, including a dietician to educate on weight loss and healthy diet; a social worker to alleviate social stressors with assistance in financial, work, and family matters; a physical therapist to help strengthen and condition the body; an occupational therapist to guide patients in choosing a job they can perform given the status of their low back pain; a recreational therapist to advise patients about the best exercises for their current condition; and, finally, a spiritual advisor to help patients keep their faith and not lose hope.

Most pain management centers are outpatient facilities, and few patients are admitted to a hospital for the purpose of relieving pain. Though inpatient treatment may be the ideal way to treat many people, insurance companies are not willing to reimburse this type of care.

At Washington University School of Medicine in St. Louis, we utilize an outpatient program, run by a psychologist and a physical therapist. A physician director will initially perform a thorough medical history and physical examination. An extensive treatment plan is created that combines the goals of reducing the pain signals coming from the body, improving the mindset of the patient experiencing pain, and enhancing his or her function. Our program follows the best recommendations of the current scientific literature by addressing the reality that the most effective treatment requires a multidisciplinary approach.

Although a pain management center is ideal, one may not be available to you, since there are a limited number of them in this country. Most of the major university-affiliated hospitals have multidisciplinary pain management centers. You can find more information about a physician located close to you by going to the Web site at www.painmed.org.

Meeting the Doctor | Strategies for successful treatment

First impressions are important in all of life, including when meeting a doctor. You will be judging the physician as he or she simultaneously analyzes you. Do your homework and learn as much as you can about the doctor before the first meeting. Ask the doctor's office to send you information, and read the Web page of the practice, if there is one.

Most doctors will want to review your medical records before meeting you, so take steps to have them sent in advance. If this is not possible, then it is helpful to bring your records with you, as well as a list of the various events related to your low back pain. (*Note: The importance of record keeping is discussed more thoroughly in chapter 12.*)

If previous radiographs (such as x-rays, CT scans, MRIs, bone scans, SPECT scans, and PET scans) have been performed, bring a copy of the radiologist's report. Find out if your new doctor wants you to bring the actual films or if the reports will be sufficient. Supplying the following information will ensure that you are relaying the most important information about your specific condition to your doctor. Write your list down and go over it in person when you and your doctor get together.

- Identify when your problem began and the circumstances surrounding it.
- List any interventions performed to try to treat the problem and the success, or lack of success, of that approach.
- If previous surgery has been performed, provide the name of the surgeon, hospital, and date of surgery. List successes and/or failures of all procedures.
- Name your primary care doctor and explain what he or she has done thus far to help you.
- List previous medications you have tried for your pain. For each one, give the date you started the medication and note how long you took it. Describe how it helped you. Record any associated effects.
- If you are continuing a medication, record who is currently prescribing it and when it was last dispensed.
- List any medications that have caused an adverse or allergic reaction. What problem(s) did it cause?
- List any active medical problems—these are problems for which you are currently seeing a physician for treatment—such as diabetes, heart disease, headaches, or arthritis.
- List previous doctors and how they tried to help your low back pain.
- List the level of your physical activity. If you attended physical therapy in the past, state what you did (exercises or modalities) and whether these exercises or modalities helped in any way.

To supply a complete health history, you must provide all relevant details, even when it may be uncomfortable to do so. If you had a bad experience with a health care procedure or provider, describe the experience. If you had a prior substance abuse problem, be candid about it. Detail the extent of the problem and what you did to correct it. Explain what actions you are taking at present to avoid relapsing in the future (for example, attending meetings of Alcoholics Anonymous or another self-help group).

If you have a current substance abuse problem, make your practitioner aware of it. A well-trained pain practitioner can help you with your pain if you are willing to obtain the necessary care for your substance abuse problem. However, if you continue to abuse drugs or alcohol, it will be very difficult for your doctor to find the correct medicines to help relieve your pain; most doctors will not work with patients under those circumstances.

First Visit | What to expect

On your first visit, you will have a complete history and physical examination. When you talk with the doctor, be candid. Give him or her your written list. Your doctor may ask many questions to clarify what you've already written down. Communicate your hopes and expectations. Be patient. Explain how your pain has affected your ability to function in activities around the house, interactions with your spouse and family, exercise, work, and sleep. Describe how your pain has affected your emotions.

The practitioner will ask some initial important questions:

Where do you feel your pain?
How intense is it?
What does it feel like (sharp, dull, burning)?
How long have the various perceptions been occurring?
What makes the pain better?
What makes it worse?

During the physical exam the doctor will assess your musculoskeletal, neurologic, and general overall health. He or she may take an x-ray of the area in your back where you are having pain and look for alignment of the spine and its relation to the pelvis. The physician will see how you walk and look at the mobility of your back. Reflexes will be tested, as will sensation and strength in specific areas.

After the history and physical, the physician will talk to you about a treatment plan. This plan should involve a discussion of your disease, such as scoliosis, spinal stenosis, degenerated discs, or herniated discs. Knowing what the disease is will help you understand the limitations it may place on your life. The doctor will also discuss potential interventions that could help you, focusing on the interventions he or she is trained to do, but the doctor should be aware of and able to discuss all options and then customize a program to fit you and your expectations. The areas of intervention to consider generally involve the following:

Functional Restoration. Do you need to work on strengthening an area of the body? Does an area need concerted treatment in order for you to have less pain and be more functional? Do you need to become more flexible? What is the level of your aerobic activity?

Coping. How are you handling your problem psychologically? Do you need help in coping with the chronic pain and its associated stresses? Do you need to have other diseases addressed, such as depression or anxiety?

Medications. What agent might help the pain you are describing? Is this a time to consider narcotic therapy?

Injections. Will injections of steroids help this pain? Is it time to implement other advanced pain management techniques, such as spinal cord stimulation?

Surgery. Does an area of the spine need to be excised or altered?

An initial treatment plan is not a "forever" approach. It can be changed. Your doctor will work with you to create a plan. You will be asked to continually assess the plan's effectiveness by detailing the various successes or failures and ultimately deciding what to keep and what to eliminate in your plan. Several visits may be necessary before you start making progress toward your goals.

Follow-up Visits | Analyzing and adjusting

Follow-up visits are scheduled regularly to reassess your pain and evaluate the course of treatment. During these visits you will want to explore the following:

- Did the treatment started at the initial visit reduce your pain? If so, how much?
- Did the treatment improve your function? If so, how?
- Are you suffering any problems related to the treatment provided? If so, what happened and how did you respond to it?

If narcotics were provided, you will be monitored to make sure you have taken the medications as prescribed. For example, a medicine for breakthrough pain should not be taken for an episode of anxiety.

Frequency of visits will vary. Usually the visits are related to your progress in managing the pain and any related treatment problems. For example, a patient who has near total relief and restored function and doesn't require narcotics may need to see the doctor only once or twice a year. A patient not benefiting from therapy who is functionally impaired and having side effects from medications may need to see the doctor daily. Most people tend to fall between these extremes.

Another area your doctor will assess is your compliance with the treatment plan. If you don't intend to follow the doctor's initial recommendations, say so outright and discuss your reasons. If the medicine is too expensive, your physician may consider similar but more affordable options. If the reason is related to a lack of motivation on your part, the physician may not want to treat you. There's no point in seeing a pain practitioner unless you are willing to make the effort to improve. If problems occur between visits, communicate with your doctor. Never change a medication regimen on your own. On the other hand, be mindful of the physician's schedule as well, and only call him or her about significant problems.

If you decide to alter your dosing of narcotics without your doctor's consent, he or she may not refill the medication or medications. This may leave you in a precarious situation in which withdrawal can occur. If a problem occurs with your medication, be truthful with your doctor; lies may return to haunt you and undermine the essential trust needed in a physician–patient relationship.

Narcotics are to be taken only by the person for whom they are prescribed. If a friend has a pain problem, refer him or her to your doctor. Do not give away any of your narcotics—sharing a narcotic is a felony. If someone in your home takes your medications for whatever reason, let your doctor know. The responsibility for your medications ultimately lies with you.

Keep track of when your medications will run out. I tell my patients to inform our office five business days before this will happen. Waiting until the last minute could cause problems: the doctor may be out of town and you may not be able to get the refill when it is needed. Mark your calendar on *the date you should call for a refill*, not on the date when your prescription runs out.

Moving to a New Location | Changing doctors

When you need to find a doctor in a new city or neighborhood, it's best to do your homework ahead of time. Some people move to a warmer climate in the hope that this will help them, only to find out that there are no physicians near their new home who are interested in managing their pain. Before planning any move, make sure you find a doctor who will be able to work with you. Ask your current doctor if he or she knows a physician in the new area. Also, you might ask him or her to write a letter to the new physician to help smooth the transition of your care.

The Internet provides the directories of many national pain organizations; these directories list physicians who manage pain and who are members of the organization. Pain organizations that may be helpful include the American Academy of Pain Medicine, the American Pain Society, and the American societies of the specialty you may want to work with (such as the American Society of Anesthesiology, for anesthesiologists). Let the organization know where you intend to move. In addition, most insurance companies will provide a list of pain management doctors in their network. Make sure you select only board-certified physicians.

Contact prospective doctors' offices to find out whether they are accepting new patients. If a doctor can see you, ask his or her office to send you printed information about the office's practice in advance, if possible.

Many physicians will send a description of their practice philosophies with welcoming packages to prospective new patients. Throughout this process, trust your instincts when deciding if a particular physician will be a good match for you.

Chapter 3
Diagnosing What's Causing Your Pain

A thorough and detailed history will help your doctor diagnose and treat your pain.

A COMPLETE AND THOROUGH EXAMINATION begins with the history of the problem. Traditionally, this is done face-to-face with the health care provider and the patient and is known as the *patient history*. This is the time to convey your goals and expectations, to determine if they are realistic and shared by everyone on your health care team.

Provide an Accurate Description | When, where, and how much

As noted in chapter 2, you will want to bring a written record of your history related to your back pain. When you meet the doctor, you will be asked when and how the pain started. Be as detailed and accurate as possible. If the pain started four years ago and you are seeking help for the first time, inform your doctor. Pain that has lingered for longer than six months is traditionally thought of as chronic in nature and is treated differently than pain that started two days ago (called acute pain). Be prepared to fully and accurately recount a fall, car accident, or work-related event that precipitated your pain.

The location of your pain is also important. Be specific. Is the pain in the low back region, radiating to your buttock or down your leg? This is known as radicular pain and can indicate a problem with the sciatic nerve or a disc in the spine. Similarly, note whether the pain wraps around from the front to the back of the body; this traditionally implies that a nerve is being irritated.

Character and intensity of pain are also important to the history process. Is the pain achy and dull, or is it more burning and throbbing? Is the pain more severe when your clothes touch it (a condition known as allodynia)? Note intensity issues, like whether the pain is worse in the morning or slowly intensifies as the day progresses. Is the pain continuous or does it come and go based upon your activity level? How does the pain impact the activities of daily living? Do you need to sit down or walk around frequently? Explain how the pain interrupts your family life, free time, work, or sexual activity. Mention any irregularities in sleep associated with discomfort. Associated factors like weakness, numbness, and increased falls or changes in bowel or bladder habits need to be shared with your physician immediately because they may indicate that you have an emergency situation. Be frank with your doctor about all these issues.

You may be asked what aggravates or worsens your pain level as well as what alleviates it or makes it better. It's important to include information about whether rest—or conversely, increased activity—has an impact on your current level of pain. Include information regarding other symptoms, such as problems with prolonged sitting or standing. Pain that worsens by sitting in a forward position for an extended period of time, for example, can indicate a problem with a herniated disc, while pain that intensifies as a result of continuous standing typically indicates spinal stenosis. You'll probably be asked what you've done to alleviate your symptoms, including the use of heat or cold packs, massage therapy, and physical therapy. It's also important to note if you've seen another health care provider, including a chiropractor or acupuncturist.

Provide Details and Family History I For an accurate diagnosis

As you share the details of your medical and surgical history with your physician, it's especially important that you include any ongoing problems with depression or anxiety. These issues can magnify pain, and your treatment will need to be adjusted accordingly. If you suffer from diabetes or cardiac disease, some medications may need to be modified in your treatment. Providing the details of your family history could help to uncover a genetic disease that may include pain among its symptoms.

Share Your Psychosocial History | Your privacy will be respected

Your psychosocial history provides vital information about how the pain is affecting you and others around you. Family dynamics change as a result of chronic pain. Understanding this and incorporating it into the plan of care is fundamental. It's natural for you to want to be circumspect about certain information, in particular a history of sexual or physical abuse or drug dependency. You may think personal information of this nature doesn't relate to treatment for back pain, but it does.

A history of substance abuse, including cigarettes, alcohol, or street drugs, needs to be addressed thoroughly so the physician can incorporate this information when planning your treatment program. If you are recovering from substance dependency, you do not want your treatment for back pain to reignite addiction problems for you. In those rare instances where a patient may be using pain to mask darker motives, such as trying to obtain prescription drugs for reasons other than their medical use, routine blood tests will reveal the truth, and legitimate physicians will refuse to administer treatment. So, if you are legitimately seeking help for your pain and you have a history of substance abuse, provide all relevant information honestly. It is best for you.

Let your doctor know of any pressure to return to work, whether the pressure comes from you, from family members, or from your workplace environment, for financial or career considerations. The more complete your personal history, the more appropriate your treatment.

Detail Your Medications | To achieve maximum benefit

As a new patient, bring a complete list of your prescription medications to your first appointment, as well as a record of your over-the-counter medications, like herbal preparations that you take to manage pain or other conditions. Although most people understand that prescription drugs can interact adversely with each other if not monitored, many people do not realize that certain herbal medications can also adversely interfere with prescription medications and potentially cause life-threatening complications as well. Studies have shown that 17 percent of the people in the United States use herbal medications, while 52 percent of Americans use vitamins or herbals.[1] If you are taking herbs or vitamins, you must share this information with your physician. Let your doctor know about any side effects you have had or continue to have from your medication. Remember, it is never wise to abruptly stop any medication without first consulting your physician. Certain medications, including antidepressants, narcotics, and antiseizure medications, need to be tapered gradually to avoid withdrawal symptoms.

Pain Scales | How much does it hurt?

Although it is not yet possible to truly measure the intensity of your pain and compare it to some standard of measurement, you will probably be asked to quantify your pain intensity on a diagram. This common diagnostic tool consists of a picture of the human body on which you mark the location and type of pain. A series of zeros may indicate a "pins and needles" feeling, while a series of Xs may indicate a sharp pain. Or, sometimes no distinction is made between the type of pain and the tool is used more simply to mark the location of any pain. It is very important to be as accurate and detailed as possible.

You may also be asked to verbally rate your pain on one of the three verbal rating pain scales: the verbal rating scale, the numerical rating scale, or the visual analogue scale (VAS). The verbal rating scale consists of several adjectives that span from no pain to extreme pain. The numerical rating scale contains a series of numbers that represent the intensity of pain experiences—your doctor may ask, "What is your pain on a scale of 1 to 10?" The visual analogue scale, perhaps the most common, displays a line, approximately 10 centimeters in length, with "no pain" labeled at one end and "worst pain imaginable" noted at the opposite end. You then place a mark on the line corresponding to your rating of pain intensity.

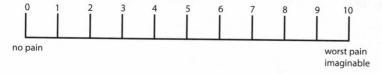

There are also more involved rating scales, including the McGill Pain Questionnaire, the Oswestry Disability Questionnaire, and the Short Form-36 Quality of Life Scale, any of which a physician may use at his or her discretion.

The Physical Examination | Getting the big picture

The physical examination of any patient, regardless of the disease process involved, continues to be one of the most important diagnostic tools doctors have at their disposal. Its purpose is multifaceted and includes developing a bond of trust between patient and physician. Your physician wants to gain an insight into the nature of the pain and the impact the pain is having on your daily life so that, together, you can map out a treatment plan that best meets your needs and goals.

The physical exam actually begins when you enter the office. An astute physician will carefully observe your mannerisms, interactions with others, pain behaviors, and gait, or walk. This provides insight into your emotional, mental, and physical well-being. The doctor will be looking for nonverbal cues—like grimacing or tearing—and pain behaviors such as vocalization—for example, moaning, grunting, and crying—or verbalization—for example, praying or swearing. He or she will also record body action that can include thrashing and rocking, rubbing, or guarding the affected area.

You may be asked to remove your clothes and put on a gown to allow the physician to carefully examine all parts of the body relevant to the problem. A systematic examination starting with the head and ending at the feet is necessary for a complete understanding of the pain process. The nurse or medical assistant will take and record your temperature, heart rate, and blood pressure, as well as your height and weight. An elevated heart rate may be an indication of your perception of pain intensity, and a difference in the blood pressure readings in your two arms—ruling out any other cause—may indicate a compression between structures in the cervical spine. The doctor will probably need to examine your skin, heart, lungs, and abdomen, in addition to the area that is causing pain.

The Cranial Examination | Observing your face

Your face and shoulders will be used to examine the twelve cranial nerves. You may be asked to stick out your tongue and squint your eyes shut or to shrug your shoulders or puff out your cheeks. These techniques, while seemingly silly to perform, help your physician differentiate between various diagnoses.

The Neck Examination | Observing your motion

Observing how you move helps your physician discover underlying pathologies. For example, your head should move naturally in relationship to your other body parts, so your doctor will ask you to walk several steps to observe your gait. You will be asked to walk on your tiptoes and then to walk on your heels. This test can signal problems with motor function. For example, a cervical cord compression may show itself in the earliest days as an alteration in a patient's ability to walk.

You will be asked to move your neck into a variety of positions including down (chin to chest), up (eyes turned upward to the ceiling), and to both sides (ear to shoulder and turning head from side to side). These tests show your range of motion. Muscle spasm, pain, and a structural problem with a disc all limit range of motion. Additionally, anatomical landmarks, including the Adam's apple (in front of the neck) and the Chassaignac's tubercle, which correspond with certain cervical discs, will be checked for abnormalities and tenderness. (The Chassaignac's tubercle is the anterior tubercle of transverse process of the sixth cervical vertebra; it is the most prominent spinal bony bump on the front of the neck and is located on both sides of the thyroid cartilage.)

The doctor may ask you to shrug your shoulders while he or she pushes down on them to test the motor strength of your neck. Next, the doctor may examine your shoulders. Uneven shoulder blades—one shoulder blade higher than the other—may signal a spinal accessory nerve dysfunction, because a dysfunctioning accessory nerve would prevent the trapezius muscle from being able to function properly. (Other causes of uneven shoulder blades include severe scoliosis.) Finally, the reflexes on the outside of your upper arm, or triceps, and in the crook of the elbow, your biceps, will likely be tested by tapping them lightly with a reflex hammer.

The Thoracic Examination | Analyzing your midback region

The thoracic examination begins with inspection of the various areas of your midback region, assessing for symmetry, muscle tone, and skin changes, such as scarring. The doctor will palpate (touch) your back to evaluate your muscle tone and range of motion. Any decreased range of motion will be documented by your physician as well as the reason for the limitation, such as pain, effort, or spasm. A decreased range of motion suggests a biomechanical problem.

The Lumbar Examination | Evaluating your low back

The majority of patients who see a doctor because of back pain complain about the low back, or lumbosacral region. The doctor must do a global inspection of this area, beginning with your gait as you enter the office. You also will be observed from behind, so the doctor can assess the curvature of the spine, to see whether it is normal. Your legs may be assessed for color or temperature changes. You may be asked to bend over at the waist, to allow the physician to assess for scoliosis (curvature of the spine) or kyphosis (a hunched back). Research has shown that lumbar scoliosis is commonly assessed on physical exam. The gluteal folds, or buttocks, and the knees should be of equal height and alignment; if they are not, the unevenness is very obvious to an experienced examiner.

Anyone who is in pain will naturally try to protect the area that is tender, but it is extremely important for you to participate fully in the physical exam so that your doctor can reach an accurate diagnosis. The physician will likely apply both soft and deeper touch to the affected area as he or she seeks to identify trigger points—those points that are especially tender. You may be asked to move in a variety of directions including bending forward, backward, and to both sides. This allows the physician to assess your range of motion (flexibility) and further pinpoint your diagnosis. Generally speaking, pain on bending forward, called flexion, indicates a disc problem, while pain on bending backward, called extension, indicates a muscle problem. Your doctor may ask you to walk on your heels or on your tiptoes, which tests the integrity of certain parts of your spine. You may be asked to squat in place, which tests general muscle strength as well as the integrity of your hip joint function. The doctor will test the reflexes on the front of your knee (patella) and on the outside of your ankle (Achilles) with a reflex hammer.

Once your doctor has examined you, you will receive a pain management plan that will include instructions for your active participation. You may be asked to observe, note, and possibly change some of your daily habits. Practical pain management tools are covered in the chapters in the next section.

Part II

Therapies from A to Z

Chapter 4
Tools for Managing Pain

Set realistic goals and believe in yourself.

THE BAD NEWS IS that chronic pain is not curable; the good news is that it is manageable. If the pain is managing you, it is time to take control. Begin by changing the way you think. Do not view your circumstances as disabling; instead, accept what you cannot change and learn to make the best of your body's new parameters. Don't mourn what you have lost; rejoice in what you have! The mind is a marvelous thing—it adapts if you let it and it adjusts quickly if you encourage it.

At this point in your life, you may be experiencing a roller coaster of emotions. You may initially feel the urge to blame others. You may feel let down by your doctors or your family because "they simply don't understand the pain" you're in. What you're feeling is understandable and normal, but it's important to remember that your pain is chronic and therefore unlikely to resolve completely. Continuing to blame others and looking for a quick fix are counterproductive behaviors. Instead, it's time to work toward a treatment plan with your physician or health care practitioner to take back control of your life and find techniques to manage the pain more effectively.

The First Steps | Analyze your pain and set some goals

The first step in gaining control over your pain is to find out what increases, or, conversely, decreases your pain level. Analyze everything, including the weather, your level of stress or tension, the activities you do each day, and how much rest you get both at night and during the day. Assessing your pain level at regular intervals, at least three times a day, is essential, because it allows you to note any patterns.

For example, after consistently analyzing your low back pain, you may notice that it's worse in the late afternoon. Furthermore, because you have tracked what you're doing in the late afternoon, you notice that long, late-afternoon meetings have become more common at work. Prolonged sitting on a hard chair is uncomfortable, even for those without chronic low back pain. Now that you've identified a time of the day when your pain is at its worst and you understand why, your next focus should be on what you can do to eliminate the discomfort.

Pain rarely remains constant. More likely, it changes in intensity or feeling by the hour, and from one day to the next. Examine your pain level closely, and accurately record it for that particular moment. Start a pain diary to record your level of pain at regular intervals. Begin by recording your pain at breakfast, lunch, dinner, and before sleeping—times that are easy to remember. Then expand. Do more than simply jotting down a number on a scale of zero to ten, registering no pain to worst pain; note your activity level during each specific time frame as well. Were you watching a movie on TV or washing the dishes? One activity is sedentary, while the other involves some form of exercise. Additional information about what you are doing to alleviate the pain should also be included. For example, what medication did you take and did it help?

Now that you've started your pain diary, you've completed the first step to bring order back to your life. After successfully tracking your pain state throughout the day for several weeks, you'll know what triggers your pain and what intensifies it. You may even have an idea about what can be done to minimize or eliminate the discomfort.

At this point, you are ready to take the next step: identify your personal objectives, like returning to the garden or playing golf in the spring. Setting goals can, in essence, give you further control over your pain. Keep your resolutions realistic and achievable. Don't plan a seven-mile

PAIN DIARY

DATE _____

BREAKFAST:

Pain Level: (1 to 10): _____

Hours & quality of sleep last night: _____

Weather: _____

Level of stress/tension: _____

Activities before breakfast: _____

Medications or steps taken to reduce pain: _____

What you ate & drank: _____

LUNCH:

Pain Level: (1 to 10): _____

Weather: _____

Level of stress/tension: _____

Activities before lunch:_____

Medications or steps taken to reduce pain: _____

What you ate & drank: _____

DINNER:

Pain Level: (1 to 10): _____

Weather: _____

Level of stress/tension: _____

Activities this afternoon: _____

Medications or steps taken to reduce pain: _____

What you ate & drank: _____

BEDTIME:

Pain Level: (1 to 10): _____

Weather: _____

Level of stress/tension: _____

Activities this evening: _____

Medications or steps taken to reduce pain: _____

Did you rest during the day? _____

What you ate & drank: _____

run until you are sure your back is up to going that distance. Your ideas also need to be measurable, which requires a method for gauging when your target has been reached. You should spell out the specific steps that need to be taken in order to accomplish your mission. Pain management calculations are "I-centered." *You are doing this for you.* You don't want to set yourself up for failure by listing too many resolutions, so start with two or three objectives at first. Avoid unrealistic expectations. Remember that we have to crawl before we can walk, and walk before we can run.

Once you identify your goals, you'll notice that accomplishing them can be physically and emotionally challenging. It's time to think positively and avoid self-defeating talk, an "emotional hook" that can talk you right out of doing the one thing you desperately want to do. An emotional hook is an irrational belief that you are going to fail—thus insuring that you will, even before you get started. Emotional hooks are disruptive to your goals. The key to overcoming them is to first identify your feelings; then analyze the potentially destructive thoughts and irrational beliefs behind them. Finally, reshape your thoughts and feelings to be more productive and less destructive.

So how can you manage negative thoughts? Write down your goals and next to them record what you are feeling about those objectives. Try to be as descriptive as possible. Are you feeling nervous, sad, or apprehensive about your intention? Next, identify how you can change this feeling. Think about a specific outcome and imagine yourself engaging in that activity. See yourself accomplishing what you want to do. Believe in its possibilities. Jot down possible obstacles, and next to each obstacle, identify the steps you must take to overcome that particular difficulty. Break it down into small steps. There is truth in the words of wisdom: Yard by yard, life is hard; inch by inch, life's a cinch; mill by mill, it's easier still. Trust in the power of small accumulated achievements.

Take Action | Pace yourself

Pacing your activities is the next step in regaining control of your pain, and subsequently of your life. When reviewing your pain diary, you may notice that your pain level is at its highest when your activity level is also high. Increasing your activity level has likely caused increased irritation or inflammation, so should you stop what you're doing and retreat to your bedroom? No!

The key is to pace yourself more effectively. Refer back to your pain diary again, if necessary. At what point during the day is your pain the greatest? Modify the activities at that time and include more opportunities for rest. Take, for example, folding clothes. If your pain level increases after 10 minutes of folding laundry (uptime), stop and rest for 10 minutes (downtime). Eventually you will be able to increase the uptime and decrease the downtime.

Your goal is not to push the body to the breaking point but to assess activities and pace them appropriately. What you want is for your back to be stronger and more flexible. Remember, you are in control of your pain, and only you can determine how you are going to manage it.

The record of activities from your pain diary is not just about time and energy devoted to an activity and downtime. It's also about listening to your body and becoming aware of the messages it is sending you. Gently stretching muscles while noting areas of tension and using deep breathing to release that tightness are just two of several techniques that will help you "listen" more effectively. When you're ready, explore exercises that are more likely to increase your uptime and decrease your downtime— walking on a treadmill or doing yoga or tai chi, for example. These two exercises are excellent because they focus on slow movements with coordinated breathing. The objective is to choose activities that empower you, which in turn will give you a greater sense of control. (See chapter 5 for a detailed discussion of exercise options.) Celebrate your successes and continue to set realistic goals.

Eat Well | Give your body what it needs

You've identified factors that increase your pain, you've set goals, and you are working toward pacing your activities. Now it's time to review good nutritional habits, which, like all the other techniques discussed thus far, are essential to overall good health. Not only does a healthy diet give your body the nutrients it needs to perform well, a healthy diet will also help you achieve and maintain your optimum body weight.

What's weight got to do with pain? Research has shown that obesity can increase the risk for degenerative joint disease, especially of the hips and knees. In addition, for people who experience chronic pain related to degenerative joint disease, the added factor of obesity can magnify their pain state.

Although this is not a book about weight loss or weight control, this factor is so important in managing—and sometimes even eliminating—pain that I want to review what science has discovered about nutrition in recent years.

We know that in order to eat a well-balanced diet, we must incorporate the basic components of the food pyramid developed by the U.S. Food and Drug Administration. Eating releases endorphins, which in turn promote a feeling of well-being and happiness. This feeling, while temporary, decreases the pain state. Healthy eating means meals with a balanced amount of protein, fat, and carbohydrates. Consuming five smaller meals rather than three large ones decreases the likelihood of overeating at one meal. Watching portion size, while not always easy, can be instrumental in preventing overeating. Eliminate "junk" or processed foods from your pantry. These add calories but do not add to your overall nutrition—in fact, sometimes just the opposite. Clearing out the junk will also make it easier to choose healthy alternatives, such as fresh fruits and vegetables. These are the first steps in regaining a healthy lifestyle.

Certain ingredients have been shown to increase pain states and therefore should be used in moderation only. These include caffeine, alcohol, monosodium glutamate (MSG), and aspartame. Caffeine, as we know, is found in most colas, coffee, tea, and chocolate. It may also be found in some over-the-counter pain medications. Alcohol causes blood vessels to become larger, which can increase the intensity of a migraine headache, for example. Listening to your body is essential in determining whether you can enjoy alcohol in moderation or whether you must eliminate it altogether. MSG, a food enhancer found in many Chinese and prepared foods, is another substance each person should assess for him- or herself, as is aspartame, the artificial sweetener in NutraSweet, Equal, and other products. Be aware of your body when you consume these ingredients. Decide whether it seems best for you to avoid them.

Research about the role vitamins and minerals play in diminishing chronic pain states is ongoing but inconclusive. Some researchers have speculated that magnesium, the B vitamins, vitamin C and E, and zinc can decrease inflammation. However, this research is not complete and lacks adequate data. People experiencing chronic pain are ready prey for anyone offering a panacea, so it's important to read labels carefully and to be cautious of any company or individual making claims that have not been tested or conclusively proven.

Although a nutritionally healthy diet can have a positive impact on your level of pain, eating only to make yourself "feel better" will ultimately have a detrimental effect. A food diary can be a helpful tool in tracking what you are eating and whether there are any diet-associated patterns to your pain.

To set healthy nutritional goals, you should know your ideal body weight, or Body Mass Index (BMI). BMI is a measure of body fat based on height and weight that applies to both adult men and women. The National Institutes of Health has devised a formula to calculate your BMI and has divided the results into four categories:

Underweight = a BMI under 18.5
Normal weight = a BMI between 18.5 and 24.9
Overweight = a BMI between 25 and 29.9
Obese = a BMI of 30 or greater

To calculate your BMI, you can use one of the many automatic calculators found on the Internet, or you can use the following formula:

$$\text{BMI} = \frac{\text{Weight in Pounds}}{\text{Height in Inches} \times \text{Height in Inches}} \times 703$$

For example, a man weighing 180 pounds with a height of 5'10" (or 70 inches) would calculate his BMI by first multiplying 70×70, which equals 4,900, then dividing 180 by 4,900, and then multiplying that number (.0367346) by 703, for a BMI of 25.82, which would place him in the overweight category. To reach the normal weight range, he would need to reduce his weight to 173.5 pounds or less.

Obesity as measured by a very high BMI has been associated with increased pain and chronic illnesses such as high blood pressure and diabetes. Reducing your BMI can reduce your risk of developing these diseases. If you find it difficult to change your nutritional habits, don't despair; instead work with a nutritionist or dietician to map out a plan that works with your lifestyle. Remember, controlling your pain is a multidisciplinary approach that requires help from various sources to succeed.

When it comes to food, choose all things in moderation. Select a diet with plenty of fruits, vegetables, and whole grains. Eliminate foods that exacerbate your pain, and reduce, or even eliminate, sugars and processed foods. Incorporate antioxidants and foods rich in vitamin A, C, and E into your diet to assist in muscle growth, reduce cell damage, and enhance recovery of compromised cells. Calcium is also important. Three to four servings a day of milk is recommended, but if milk disagrees with you, consider nondairy calcium-rich foods like beans, broccoli, greens, salmon, fortified juices, and almonds.

Exercise | Move your body

Any chapter on tools for managing pain must include exercise. But if you're like most patients, when I say the word "exercise," you cringe. You may even catch yourself thinking, "I can't possibly exercise, I already hurt enough." The fear of further injury is a common one. But it's a misconception that complete bed rest will return you to your baseline level of functioning and that the pain will resolve on its own without further intervention. To improve mobility and flexibility, light stretching, conditioning, and strengthening exercises are essential. Target the muscles that strengthen the spine and support the bones and joints as a first step to reducing pain.

You can begin slowly by gradually introducing more movement into your life. Take the stairs instead of the elevator. Park your car farther away from your destination in a parking lot. Walk to the neighborhood store, if possible.

When you are ready, you may want to consider joining a gym. There, too, it is suggested that you start slowly, increasing your workout as you're able to. Working out with a professional, while not required, ensures that you are exercising correctly and decreases the likelihood that you will injure yourself further. Also, a trainer can help you map out an exercise plan that meets your individual needs and goals. Research has shown that exercise, when used properly, can decrease your perception of pain, return you to work faster, and allow you to recover your baseline level of functioning more quickly. Research has even shown that regular exercise can help prevent osteoporosis and potential fractures that could result in more pain. Avoiding exercise for even a week or two can cause the back to lose muscle tone and strength and result in muscle spasms with pain from even the mildest kind of manipulation, like bending over to pick up a paper clip. (Exercise is covered more fully in chapter 5.)

Hot and Cold | When to use which

Applying moist heat before and after exercise will diminish muscle spasms and decrease inflammation. Heat allows for an increased blood flow to the site of pain, which in turn promotes decreased inflammation and joint stiffness. You must be careful to avoid the risk of burn: don't leave heat on an area for longer than 15 minutes. Heat can be applied in a variety of forms: take a warm shower, relax in a whirlpool or hot tub, loll in a warm bath, or apply a heat pack or moist heating pad or a moist, warm towel. Consult your physician before using heat therapy, especially if you suffer from poor circulation or other illnesses.

Cold therapy, whether through ice or a cold pack, can also be beneficial in diminishing muscle spasms. Never apply ice directly to the skin without a barrier, as this can cause serious skin damage and potentially increase your pain level. Some research suggests that alternating heat and cold applications can maximize the benefit of each. Many physicians and health care providers subscribe to the RICE formula for treating *pain caused by injury*: Rest, Ice, Compression, and Elevation. Rest the injured area temporarily; apply ice in a pack to the affected area in 20 minutes on, 2 minutes off, increments; apply a firm compression bandage, such as an Ace wrap, to minimize swelling; and elevate the affected area, also to minimize swelling.

Sleep Well | Find a good position

Odd as it may seem, another "tool" in the pain management arsenal—identifying a comfortable sleeping position—is not as straightforward as it appears. Although bed rest is not recommended for an extended time, adequate rest can help with pain. There are two generally accepted positions for patients with chronic back pain: lying on one's side with hips and knees bent at a 90-degree angle and a small pillow placed between the legs; and lying on one's back with legs slightly elevated by a pillow under the knees. The second position normally works best for people already accustomed to sleeping on their backs. If you normally sleep on your stomach, you may find these preferred positions difficult and, at first, un-comfortable. If you simply cannot avoid sleeping on your stomach, place a pillow under it, which allows the spine to straighten out, decreasing the pressure on the spine.

Getting out of bed safely requires making a smooth transition from lying down to standing up, with no sudden movements. First, turn on the side from which you will be rising and slowly work your way to the edge of the bed. While keeping your back straight, use your lower arm and the palm of your hand to slowly push yourself to the sitting position. This technique allows your legs to naturally fall over the bed and gently touch the floor. From here, you will be able to transition from sitting to standing. Consider using an assistive device—a cane or walker—if you feel unsteady on your feet.

Think Good Thoughts | Develop and maintain a good attitude

Perhaps the most important tool for adapting to a lifestyle with pain is a flexible attitude. Attitudes are learned beliefs and behaviors that can be the result of cultural influences. In general, they shape your thoughts and actions on a daily basis without your being aware of their influence.

Attitude becomes a problem when it impedes normal growth and development. Take the person who continues to smoke despite a diagnosis of lung cancer. He feels that stopping is not going to change the diagnosis, so "Why bother?" True, quitting isn't going to make the lung cancer go away, but it will improve his overall physical and psychological health. A person who believes that he or she has no control over the events in life may very well continue to engage in unhealthy behaviors.

Two unhealthy attitudes common in chronic pain patients are "learned helplessness" and anger and hostility. Learned helplessness is based on the notion that after repeatedly doing something you know causes pain, you eventually stop doing all similar things for fear that they too will inflict the level of pain associated with the original. For example, you may refuse to fully engage in physical therapy because you're afraid it will trigger worse pain. Overcoming learned helplessness is important in gaining control of your pain.

Anger and hostility are emotional cancers that eat away at your overall health and your immune system responds accordingly. If you allow yourself to dwell on the negative, your immune system may follow your lead, possibly making you vulnerable to multiple potential disorders, including chronic pain.

A healthy attitude starts with optimism. Research has shown that optimism can boost the natural immune system. Pessimists, on the other hand, see every life event as something negative. They are more likely to expect negative events to happen to them because they've happened before. Pessimistic individuals tend to be in poor health and suffer from depression. It's good to remember that attitudes are not rigid and unchangeable and that developing a healthy attitude, while it requires work, will benefit you forever.

Humor is an important component of a healthy attitude. It's all too easy to become so preoccupied with pain that you fail to find humor in anything. Watching a funny movie or sharing a joke with a friend can reinforce a healthy mind-body connection. Anything that gives you a good-natured laugh will make you feel better at some level. Searching for the humor in life can revitalize the soul and release endorphins, and endorphins, in turn, can diminish the perception of pain.

Start with small steps to achieve positive thoughts and develop healthy behaviors that will carry you into the next phase of reclaiming your life and managing your pain. Holding onto negative attitudes is counterproductive and can depress your mind and spirit. Examine your conscious and unconscious feelings and remember: attitude is a choice, and, therefore, you have the control to define your attitude.

Understanding your pain and incorporating the tools mentioned above is an excellent start to taking control. However, there will be times when, in spite of how hard you try or the successes you achieve, stressors will knock you off course, causing you to question your ability to make progress. If this happens, it's up to you to overcome this crisis in self-confidence by taking control of your thoughts and not letting them control you.

Consider this scenario as an example. Perhaps you have been making steady progress and enjoying some successes; your attitude is good and your pain is becoming more manageable. But one afternoon, while visiting the zoo with your grandchildren, you have a tremendous flare of pain. A flare of pain is not an uncommon setback, but having a plan to deal with it can mean the difference between retreating to your bed for days—or weeks—and simply adjusting your goals. Being prepared can minimize the frustration you will feel. Your "crisis plan" should include a list of the options available and the techniques you have found to be helpful in dealing with new or intensified pain.

Your options for a trip to the zoo might include requesting a handicapped parking spot, riding a tourmobile rather than walking long distances, and bringing along your medication. Your options for everyday life might include reserving a temporary parking spot closer to the door at work or using a motorized cart at the grocery store, for the short term. If taking a soothing bath with scented soap relaxes you, then do it. If being outside in the warm sunshine is comforting, spend time sitting outdoors. Focus on the relaxation techniques you have found to be helpful; use breathing exercises such as inhaling and exhaling deeply and slowly. The key is not to overwhelm your body when it is already under stress; instead, redirect your thoughts and actions away from the pain.

Chapter 5
Exercise for Treating Pain

🌱 *with Elizabeth Pegg Frates, M.D.*

Move to improve. The benefits are priceless.

Note: Check with your physician before doing any exercise. In order to avoid injury, people with some specific conditions should never perform certain exercises.

EXERCISE IS IMPORTANT FOR everyone and especially important for those working to minimize their back pain. The benefits of exercise are extensive. In fact, almost every organ and tissue in our bodies benefits from exercise—including the brain, muscles, heart, lungs, bones, connective tissue, and even our cells. That's right, our cells—our muscle cells and our brain cells, which are two examples that will be explored in more detail later in the chapter. The benefits of exercise are widespread and interconnected. It can help the whole body function at a higher level of wellness.

This chapter provides a solid foundation in exercise basics and a road map for how back pain patients can be more physically active. The three essential elements of an exercise routine are aerobic activity, stretching, and strengthening.

One of the most important things you can do for yourself is talk to your doctor about exercise. Exercise is safe only after your doctor gives you medical clearance to proceed. Someone with an acute severe disc herniation requiring surgery, for example, should avoid exercise. However, for the vast majority of chronic back pain patients, the back pain is not the limiting factor with exercise. Rather, it is the patient's overall poor conditioning that may be problematic. A patient's heart, lungs, and overall health need to be evaluated before a physician recommends exercise to a specific patient.

The general guidelines and information on exercise in this chapter can serve as a starting point for your conversation with your own doctor in order to develop the exercise program that is right for you.

Medical researchers have conducted many scientific studies over the years to see whether exercise helps people with back pain. A comprehensive review article on this subject was written by Dr. James Rainville, a physiatrist at the New England Baptist Hospital in Boston, Massachusetts. He and his colleagues concluded that "most studies have observed improvements in global pain ratings after exercise programs, and many have observed that exercise can lessen the behavioral, cognitive, affect, and disability aspects of back pain syndromes."[1]

Definitions | Getting the lay of the land

When people say *exercise,* what do they mean? Many people think of jogging, biking, basketball, tennis, soccer, and mountain climbing when they hear the term exercise. Sports as exercise can be intimidating to people who feel they couldn't possibly "exercise" unless they were in excellent physical condition. The thought of playing soccer or jogging is not appealing to most patients suffering from back pain. However, walking, balancing on and sitting on a therapeutic big rubber ball, performing leg lifts, and stretching are all forms of physical activity that are good for your body. These activities fall into the broad category of physical activity, which is defined as any bodily movement. In contrast, the term exercise refers to a subset of physical activity that is planned and structured.

Lifestyle exercise is a term that is gaining in popularity and importance. This term refers to physical activity that you do in the course of your daily life, such as taking the stairs instead of the elevator, gardening, sweeping the floor, washing the car, walking the dog, walking from the parking lot to the store, or biking to work (for those "going green"). For people with back pain, the first physical activity goal might be to engage in lifestyle exercise and find ways to incorporate movement into the day. When you think of exercise, think of movement and being physically active. Don't forget about lifestyle exercise.

You may be wondering why you should be thinking or even reading about exercise when you have back pain. The answer is that physical activity may reduce your back pain. In days gone by, bed rest was considered a treatment for back pain. However, now we realize that, in most cases, bed rest can be helpful for a day or two, but after that it has the potential to make matters worse by causing deconditioning, muscle atrophy, and decreased flexibility. There is a cycle to inactivity. The less you move around, the weaker you become, and the less you want to move around. Movement is the way to break the inactivity cycle.

What can physical activity do for you? For your brain, it can improve your mood, decrease anxiety, increase concentration and focus, and even decrease the likelihood of dementia. In a book titled *Spark: The Revolutionary New Science of Exercise and the Brain*, Dr. John Ratey explains in laymen's terms how routine exercise acts as an antidepressant similar to prescription medicines that increase the levels of the neurotransmitters serotonin and norepinephrine. Dr. Ratey also shares the results of research demonstrating that exercise raises levels of a neurotransmitter that is involved in relaxation and is also the active agent in many antianxiety medications. It has been demonstrated in research that exercise increases brain-derived neurotrophic-factor (BDNF), which helps the brain create new synapses and make more connections. Dr. Ratey describes BDNF as "fertilizer" for the neurons (brain cells). That is an example of how exercise actually affects our brain cells, called neurons. We now have strong scientific evidence that physical activity has powerful effects on the brain and neurons.

Muscles also gain from physical activity, in more ways than one. Getting stronger is an obvious benefit that allows you to participate in more activities. However, physical activity also affects the inner workings of the muscles. Research shows that muscle exposed to regular exercise or trained muscle has different metabolic properties than untrained or deconditioned muscle. Scientific studies demonstrate that muscle cells alter their metabolic activity after routine exercise training such that the muscles increase their glycogen levels, which allows them to store more glucose. In addition, exercise increases the levels of glucose transporter 4 (GLUT4), which helps transport glucose (sugar) from the bloodstream into the muscles for storage.[2] These metabolic changes allow the body to function with greater insulin sensitivity, which helps control blood sugars and, in turn, helps control and may even prevent diabetes.

Stretching exercises, which are another type of physical activity, affect muscles by lengthening and loosening the tendons that attach muscles to bone. Tight and stiff muscles limit range of motion. Stretching the muscles decreases this tightness and increases flexibility. In turn, increased flexibility improves range of motion around a joint, can allow someone to participate in more physical activity, and also helps avoid future injuries.

Exercise has been shown to help prevent and manage many diseases including osteoporosis, heart disease, high blood pressure, high cholesterol, type 2 diabetes, metabolic syndrome, and obesity. It has even been shown to help prevent some cancers, including colon cancer. In fact, there is evidence that exercise reduces what physicians call "all-cause mortality," which basically means dying from all different causes.[3]

It sounds too good to be true. However, the power of exercise has been appreciated and discussed for hundreds of years. It is not until recently that we have had the science to back up our beliefs and personal experiences. That is why the American College of Sports Medicine and the American Medical Association started a physical activity campaign titled "Exercise Is Medicine" (www.exerciseismedicine.org). There is a push to make physical activity one of the vital signs that are checked each time you have a routine visit with a health care provider. Your level of physical activity would be checked just like your weight, blood pressure, and temperature. Physical activity is critical to good health and written exercise prescriptions are the wave of the future. "Physical activity adds years to your life and life to your years."[4]

At this point you might be saying, "That's great, but how will physical activity help to get rid of my pain?" The answer has many parts to it. For example, if you are overweight, that excess weight is putting stress on your body and may be contributing to your back pain. The best way to lose weight is to eat less and exercise more. In addition, strengthening the muscles of your back and those in your core abdominal area will help support your back and therefore protect your back. Strong muscles can help prevent acute flare-ups of back pain. Exercise may even help you feel less pain with activity.

Maybe you've heard of something called a *runner's high*. The good news is that it doesn't just come from running. It is the pleasant feeling a person can experience after engaging in a session (at least 20 minutes) of physical activity. It is thought to be created by the release of the body's own natural opioids, called endorphins. In fact, some people who are addicted to narcotics go through a drug rehabilitation program and substitute addictions—instead of being addicted to drugs, they become addicted to exercise. They lose weight, get physically fit, improve their health, and still get that "high" feeling.

There is a positive cycle of exercise that is important for back pain patients. Many people with back pain just do not feel like being physically active. This feeling of inertia is often caused by weeks or years of inactivity, contributing to deconditioning, weight gain, stiffness, isolation, loneliness, pain, and possibly even depression. By initiating movement, you can start a positive cycle—the physical activity cycle. The more you move around, the better you feel, and the more you want to move around. Getting fresh air on a walk around the neighborhood, visiting with friends that you meet on a walk in a park, or the sense of accomplishment you get from planting flowers in your garden are all positive reinforcements that will encourage you to be more active. Focusing on the positive is key with exercise, as it is with most aspects in our lives. There is a lot of truth to the saying, "What we appreciate, appreciates." If we appreciate the benefits of exercise, we will value them and strive to achieve them.

With respect to the "dose" of physical activity that is required to attain health benefits, remember one important point. Some is better than none. The United States Health and Human Services Department released physical activity recommendations for American adults in October 2008. These are the first federal guidelines on physical activity, and they can be found online at www.health.gov/paguidelines. In general, it is recommended that adults accumulate 150 minutes of physical activity each week. This amounts to about a half an hour five days a week, but you do not need to break it up this way. Depending on your schedule, you could do 20 minutes six days a week and 30 minutes one day a week if you want to take a walk every day at lunch and only have 20 minutes to do so.

These recommendations are meant as guidelines and are not meant to scare people who are currently inactive or sedentary. In fact, in the 632-page report from the U.S. Department of Health and Human Services (which is available online at the same Web site), it is stressed that going from no physical activity in a week to even one hour of physical activity a week (which is less than 10 minutes a day) provides health benefits. A little physical activity goes a long way for your health. One hundred fifty minutes a week might be an intimidating, unattainable concept right now, but 10 minutes a day is most likely a manageable goal.

If getting moving seems beyond your reach at this time, there are things you can do to help you become more physically active, including physical therapy, occupational therapy, vocational therapy, and learning about proper posture and body mechanics.

Physical Therapy | A medical approach to exercise

I refer patients to physical therapy (PT) to help them learn how to function better and become more physically active. PT is a form of organized, prescribed exercise targeted at specific parts of the body and is taught and implemented by a licensed physical therapist. Its core principles are to increase function and strength while at the same time improving quality of life. A good physical therapy program will offer not a cure for low back pain, but rather the tools to better manage the pain. PT can help prevent further back pain episodes and may even help reduce the pain. For more information about physical therapy, speak to your physician or go to the Internet. The American Physical Therapy Association (APTA) hosts its own Web site at www.apta.org.

Just as during your first visit to a physician, your first meeting with a physical therapist starts with a detailed history and physical exam. He or she will record both what you say and what he or she observes about your limitations. The physical therapist will be aware that any part of dysfunction in the musculoskeletal system below the belly button may lead to low back pain.

Once the physical therapy assessment is complete, the physical therapist will work with you to map a plan of care that meets your goals and needs. He or she will demonstrate exercises that will help you meet these goals and probably schedule repeat sessions where you will be able to practice these exercises under supervision. You may be asked to continue the exercises at home. After some time, you should notice improvement in your physical performance. The therapist may also utilize heat and cold application, which has been shown to reduce inflammation, relax sore muscles, stimulate tissue healing, and improve blood flow. Other methods or techniques used by physical therapists to help reduce pain include ultrasound, massage, and mild electrical stimulation.

Your physician may ask the physical therapist to try to "shock" your nerves to health by using Transcutaneous Electrical Nerve Stimulation (TENS). TENS works by changing your perception of pain. More specifically, the mild electrical stimulation you feel when you use a TENS unit overrides the pain signals coming from your area of discomfort. As the TENS unit blocks pain signals, you will notice a decrease in your pain level. TENS uses an electrical current applied through a series of electrodes placed on the skin to stimulate the large-diameter sensory fibers. Although the frequency of the stimulation pattern can alternate between low and high, the most commonly prescribed models will be low frequency.

Generally, the TENS unit is a small portable device that has two to four "leads" that produce low voltage electrical current. The electrodes are placed around the painful area, in this case, the low back region. Wires are attached to the electrodes, and then, through a small, battery-powered machine, a small electrical current is passed between them. Most patients describe the sensation as a mild tingling. The electrical sensation can be adjusted by using the high frequency/low intensity mode. You should continue to adjust until a buzzing or tingling sensation is felt, using the machine in 20- to 30-minute increments. If there is no noticeable improvement in the level of pain experienced, the therapist can move the electrodes around until trigger points can be identified. If pain is usually felt in the normal distribution of a nerve pathway, you should place an electrode directly over that area.

There are minimal or no side effects from long-term use of TENS. Mild skin irritation from the adhesive on the electrodes sometimes occurs, and the physician can suggest something to minimize this problem. If you have an implanted pacemaker, you may not be able to use a TENS device. There are no documented studies showing damage from the electrical current. Like most of the therapies suggested in this book, TENS should be used in conjunction with other techniques. Most physical therapy and rehabilitation facilities use TENS units. Units are available for home use, but trying it in a professional environment first, before purchasing a TENS unit, is advisable.

The therapeutic response to physical therapy is varied and can result in everything from overall improvement at best, to exacerbation of the symptoms in cases where the exercises are improperly performed or are not performed at all. However, it's important to note that patients who stay active are far more likely to improve than those who don't move around regularly to get their daily "dose" of physical activity.

Occupational Therapy | Focusing on activities of daily living

Physical therapists tend to focus on the lower extremities while occupational therapists tend to focus on the upper extremities and activities of daily living like dressing, eating, and bathing. It is possible that you may benefit from occupational therapy (OT), especially if you have not been active for many months and your deconditioned, stiff muscles are making activities like personal grooming a challenge for you. The occupational therapist will help you work on strengthening and stretching your arm muscles with the goal of increasing your functional capacity (your ability to function on a daily basis). This might be especially important if you are suffering from neck and upper back pain in addition to low back pain.

Vocational Rehabilitation | Getting back to work

Another type of therapy is vocational therapy, and vocational therapists help people get back to work by addressing whatever is limiting their ability to perform their job. Getting back to work and feeling productive is an important goal for many low back pain patients. Physiatrists can help determine if you are ready to go back to work based on individual medical assessments. If you are not ready to go back, you may benefit from physical therapy, occupational therapy, or a functional restoration program that is designed to increase your strength and flexibility with the goal of getting you back to work and restoring function (hence the name, functional restoration). Some people view functional restoration programs as back pain boot camps. The term "boot camp" alarms most people and excites very few. However, functional restoration programs can be life altering for many. If you are trying to get back to work but do not feel ready physically, then speak to your physician about a functional restoration program.

If you are back at work, you might benefit from an evaluation of your worksite. A vocational therapist can do this. The therapist will examine your workstation and check that it is "back healthy." He or she would pay special attention to:

- the location of your keyboard in relation to your computer
- the height of your chair in relation to the top of your desk

By making sure your workstation is set up properly, the vocational therapist will help you maintain good sitting posture and body mechanics throughout your work day.

If your job requires more mobility than a desk job would, a vocational therapist can evaluate your body mechanics as you load, lift, stack, and move around. The therapist can offer suggestions as to how you can complete your job while maintaining proper body mechanics and good posture. You might need to have limitations put on your work duties, depending on your personal situation. Your physician and therapist can help you determine what will work best for you at your job. In certain cases, changing responsibilities at work or even changing jobs is the best option. There is a lot to consider when making decisions about your work. It all depends on the specifics of your problem and the details of your job.

The Importance of Posture | One of Mom's favorites

One of the fundamental practices in physical therapy, occupational therapy, and vocational therapy is observing posture. After decades of poor posture, complaints of low back pain are not unusual. Poor posture causes strain and stress on the various ligaments, facets, and discs of the lower back, all of which can lead to chronic pain.

Do you remember your mother saying, "Stand up straight" or "Stop sitting all hunched over"? In this case, mom really did know best. Poor posture can cause pain and fatigue. Posture can be divided into two categories: static and dynamic. Static posture is the position your body is in when it is still, as in standing, sitting, or lying down. Dynamic posture refers to a body in motion, as when you are walking, bending, or lifting. Examining both postures can help you identify unhealthy habits—the first step to improving them.

Developing a proper back exercise program starts with evaluating your posture habits. A good way to do this is to stand sideways in front of a full-length mirror exactly the way you stand normally. Be sure not to "try to stand straight"—it's important for you to see how you really stand. Now, ask yourself some basic questions.

- Are your knees locked or bent?
- Is your waistline level with your low back?
- Are your shoulders rounded or slumped over?
- Are your head and neck tilted forward away from your shoulders?

Your knees should be reasonably straight, with only a slight bend, and not locked into place. There should be a mild inward curvature in the lumbar region of your back and your stomach should be slightly tucked in. Good posture begins with shoulders that are in a straight line with your torso, the main part of your body. It is also important that your head be centered over the top of the chest in a leveled position and your neck should show only a slight curvature.

Adopting healthy standing habits doesn't happen overnight. It takes time and attention, a process made easier when you keep in mind that you are taking control of your pain and making healthy changes not just for tomorrow but for a lifetime. It may be easier to practice a healthy standing position against a wall. Practice performing a pelvic tilt, which requires you to move the small of your back toward the wall while at the same time tilting your pelvis forward. It may sound complicated, but once you get the hang of it, it will be easy. Lining up your pelvis with the rest of your body makes walking easier on the spine. Remember, keep your knees slightly bent and not locked into position. If you are looking for visual images of good posture, you can search the Internet and find many good examples.

If you find that you have to stand for prolonged periods of time, a footrest can be a beneficial tool. Alternating feet on the footrest can decrease the strain on the facet joints in the low back. Also, when standing for a prolonged period of time, avoid bending or leaning over, which causes uneven alignment of the low back. For women, wearing high heels increases the curvature of the low back and places it at greater risk for muscle strain and fatigue. Wearing a heel that allows for an even distribution of support, like a flat or a platform heel, will lessen this stress factor.

Walking | A powerful weapon when used properly

Just as proper standing habits are important, walking habits can impact the overall health of your back. Again, take that full-length mirror and walk in front of it.

- Do you walk with your stomach punched out or your head looking down at the ground?
- Does your abdomen protrude farther than the rest of your body?
- Do you walk stiffly or, conversely, are you a victim of "loose" walking?
- Do you have one of the worst walking habits, the heel-pounding walk?

Walking with the stomach out increases the forward arch of your lower back, causing the pelvis to tilt in an unnatural fashion. If your abdomen protrudes farther than the rest of your body, work to change this habit by keeping your hips and your lower back in a stable neutral position. This will involve incorporating a slight pelvic tilt as you walk. This small adjustment will cause your pelvis to line up with the rest of your body and make walking easier on you and your spine.

Head-forward walking involves looking down at the ground as you walk. When you do this, you are placing your chest in a sunken position, thus increasing the stress on your neck, shoulders, and lower back. Not only is this bad for your spine, but ultimately it can cause poor breathing and decreased endurance. Instead, focus your attention on allowing your head and trunk to be naturally upright. Do not allow your head to bend forward, backward, or to either side. Instead focus your head on the events directly in front of your face.

Wobbling and flailing the arms characterize "loose" walking. This is most commonly seen in people with joint instability or muscle weakness.

Medical attention can determine the reason for it and physical therapy can help stabilize it. Conversely, "stiff" walking is often the result of an individual's fear of causing further harm to his or her back. This kind of walk causes muscles to work harder and creates a never-ending body contraction that, in effect, increases the likelihood of re-injury.

The heel-pounding walk is characterized by a thudding sound with every step. This sends shock waves from the foot up the leg and right into the spinal joints. People prone to this type of walking are often in a hurry, emotionally upset, barefoot, or wearing hard spiked heels. In order to reduce the amount of pounding, focus on gently placing your foot to the ground; striving for a quieter and smoother flow in your walk; imagining your head and neck to be completely "light"; and allowing yourself to relax and decrease muscle tension. Finally, remember that your choice of shoes makes a difference.

Sitting | A necessity

Many of our usual activities require a great deal of sitting, and sitting can cause more strain on the low back than standing. If proper body mechanics are not utilized, prolonged sitting can cause muscles to tire quickly. This can lead to slouching in the seat in order to alleviate the tired, sore muscles. Slouching, in turn, causes the center of gravity to shift forward. The result is that the pelvis rotates backward, placing your lumbar (or low) back in an awkward position. This posture causes the disc in your low back to bear the entire weight of your upper body unevenly.

To start your sitting evaluation, sit in a chair that is typical for you and exaggerate your normal "comfortable position." Remember, let go and relax. It may help to do it in front of that same full-length mirror for better visualization. Note whether you have any of the following poor posture characteristics:

- slumping
- tense sitting
- crossed legs

Slumped posture occurs when your lower back is rounded out, your chest is sunk in, your upper back is leaning forward, and your neck is arched backward in order to keep your head level. Slumping greatly increases the pressure in your low back. In this position, the joints in the mid- and upper portion of your neck are crammed together and the muscles in your neck and shoulders are overused. Prolonged sitting in this position will ultimately cause difficulty in straightening up into an erect position.

Tense sitting refers to long-term sitting with prolonged tension in your muscles, most likely because your lower back is unsupported. Tense posture typically occurs from stress, and many people are not aware of their tension until it is brought to their attention, as with biofeedback.

Crossed legs, a common sitting posture for women, can be a culprit in low back pain. For short periods of time, this position is comfortable and allows your muscles to relax. However, if you maintain it for an extended period of time, you lose the support of your muscles—they get too relaxed—and you will compensate by adopting either the slumped or tense sitting position.

One of the worst sitting "habits"—although undetectable in a mirror—is sitting too long, something that is hard to avoid in this age of computers. Unfortunately, our bodies are not designed to be in one position for a prolonged period of time. Sitting for even an hour without adequate rest breaks places increased pressure on the joints and discs in the low back.

Don't despair. If you are guilty of poor sitting posture, you can correct it. Because your pelvis affects the entire position of your low back, start there. To position your pelvis correctly, move your tailbone back as far as possible in your chair with your upper body tilting forward. Tucking your pelvis into the back of your chair will bring your body into an upright position. Experiment with adjusting your pelvis until it feels comfortable for you. Keep your head, chest, and pelvis properly aligned to keep stressful pressure off your back. Placing a small footstool under your feet (the ones with a slant are best) will cause you to lift your knees approximately to hip level, thus putting your pelvis into a healthy position. If you like to sit on the edge of your chair, you should keep your knees lower than your hips and move your legs wider apart than what is considered normal, with one foot positioned forward and the other farther back on the floor.

Correct body mechanics is only one piece of the puzzle; getting a chair that properly maintains your low back is another. A good chair holds your spine in its natural shape for as long as you sit in it. Although more expensive, an office chair that offers lumbar support can make the difference between sore tired muscles and muscles that can help you for hours each day. Avoid a chair you sink into, as this can cause muscles in the low back to compensate for the lack of support. If possible, get a chair that has armrests, because they decrease tension and fatigue in the neck and shoulders.

If you have an office chair that doesn't offer support, you can still improve your sitting position and minimize tension and fatigue. Place a rolled up towel or small pillow across the small of your back in order to maintain that natural curvature of the spine. Take breaks and move around. Most of us get caught up in our tasks and discover that before long we've been sitting at a desk or computer for several hours without changing our position. Although it's difficult to interrupt work, especially when faced with deadlines, frequent stretching will rejuvenate your lower back and allow you to be more productive in the long run.

Proper Lifting | Keep it light; do it right

Lifting and bending are the two everyday movements that are the most common causes of low back strain. One of the biggest mistakes you can make when performing these movements is placing your feet too close together. Feet closer than shoulder-width apart result in poor leverage and instability. When feet are positioned wider apart, they remind you to bend at the hips, not the waist, and keep the back relatively straight.

When you lift, it's important to keep the object as close as possible to the body. When picking up an object from the floor, keeping your elbows and forearms in contact with the insides of your thighs will make you more stable and shift the weight from the spine to the legs. Lifting objects that are too heavy or carrying an imbalanced load can be rough on even the healthiest of backs, resulting in strain and causing pain.

An imbalanced load results when something heavy is carried in one hand while the other hand carries nothing. (Travelers beware!) If necessary, divide your load so that equal pressure is applied to both sides of your body. If the load is simply too heavy, utilize a cart or make multiple trips. The additional time is well worth it when you consider the possibility of a back injury. It is also advisable to *push* a heavy object rather than *pull* it because pushing places less strain and stress on your lower back.

Avoid twisting when lifting. (Snow shovelers beware!) Twisting places a great deal of pressure and stress in the structures of the low back, which can potentially cause disc herniations or other injuries. Always follow standard lifting guidelines. In general, women can lift a load of 30 to 35 pounds, while men can typically lift 50 to 60 pounds. If you need to lift any object heavier than this, ask for help or use a cart or dolly.

Stretching | The cornerstone for healthy back motion and protection

Stretching is one of the most important physical activities a person with back pain can do for him- or herself. It is a critical element of maintaining a healthy back. Check in with your physician before starting any type of stretching routine, and discuss any limitations you might have. Your physician might prescribe physical therapy for you. As mentioned previously, a physical therapist can help you get started and teach you the proper methods of stretching. After a few sessions with a physical therapist, you will receive a home stretching program, which you can and should do at home. It is recommended that you stretch at least three days a week for 15 minutes each session. If you can stretch seven days a week, that is even more helpful. There is no harm in stretching, if it is done properly.

While stretching, the cardinal rule is to avoid bouncy and jerky movements. In fact, it is recommended that you hold the stretch position for 30 seconds. This helps avoid injury and allows for optimal stretching. If this seems unattainable at first, work on holding the position for 5 seconds and slowly increase the time as you become more accustomed to the stretch and you become more flexible.

Do not hold your breath as you hold a stretch. Breathe comfortably and slowly. During stretching you want to be relaxed, and deep breathing helps your body reach a state of relaxation. After each stretch, rest for a few seconds and take a few deep breaths. Then, proceed to the next stretch.

How far do you stretch the muscle? This is a common question for the novice stretcher. The answer is to listen to your body and to trust the signals it sends you. Stretching is not meant to be a painful experience. The key is to stretch to the point where you can "feel the stretch," meaning the point at which you sense your muscle being lengthened. Basically something feels different in your muscle as you stretch it. It should feel different, but not painful. Hold the stretch at this point, continue to breathe, and start to count, at least up to five. Initially, you may only be able to count to three (one–one thousand, two–one thousand, three–one thousand). That is okay. You will work up to five slowly. The key is not to bounce the muscle in and out of the stretch. Remember to relax, breathe, go slowly, avoid abrupt, jerky movements, and simply try to enjoy the stretch.

There are several different stretches you can perform to help increase flexibility in your back. Discuss the specific stretches with your physician because certain exercises can be dangerous for patients with specific conditions. For example, patients with osteoporosis need to be careful with flexion (bending forward) exercises, as they can cause fractures.

Below you will find a list of stretches that may be helpful to back pain patients, depending on their condition. If possible, stretch from head to toe. Stretch opposing muscle groups equally, meaning stretch those muscles that flex a joint as well as the muscles that extend a joint. For example, stretch those neck muscles that help you move your neck forward and those that help you move your neck backward. Don't forget to rest in between stretches. Take a few deep breaths while you rest.

When stretching muscles there are six different motions to consider: forward flexion, backward extension, left-side bending, right-side bending, left rotation, and right rotation.[5] Most of the stretches listed below can be done sitting or standing. Some of them are performed while lying down. These are simply suggestions. Use them as a guide and a reference to start a conversation about stretching with your physician or therapist. Your own stretching routine might vary from the one described here.

Neck Stretches

Bend neck forward (moving chin down toward chest). Rest. Bend neck backward (moving chin up to sky). Rest. Bend neck to the left (moving left ear toward left shoulder). Rest. Bend neck to the right (moving right ear to right shoulder). Rest. Rotate the neck to the left by gently looking to the left while keeping your head eye level. Rest. Do the same for the right side.

Arm/Shoulder Stretches

Raise arms above your head. Keeping your head, shoulders, and knees parallel while standing, place arms shoulder level and push away from your body while reaching forward, in front of you. Rest and then reach arms back behind you. Remember, hold these stretches for at least 5 seconds or as long as possible working up to 30 seconds.

Back Stretches

Flexion

Lean forward, flexing your back. This can be done while sitting in a chair, moving your chest to your knees, and reaching for the ground. It can also be done standing with knees straight, bending at the waist, bringing your chest to your legs, and reaching for the floor. Hold the stretch for as long as you can, aiming for 30 seconds. When you first attempt this exercise, you may not come close to touching the ground (sitting or standing). Make a mental note as to how close you are to the floor, 2 feet or 2 inches. After a few weeks of regular stretching, you are bound to see an improvement.

Back flexion is a range of motion that is often measured in the physician's office. You can ask your physician to measure your back flexion before starting the stretching program and then again after a few weeks of regular stretching. This is one way to demonstrate a concrete change with numbers. If you are a goal-oriented, numbers type of person, it might be motivating to strive to change the numbers and increase your range of motion with back flexion.

Extension

Bend backwards, extending your back. If possible, place your hands at the small of your back, with palms touching your body and lean backward into your hands. This back extension movement can be done standing or modified for sitting. It should not be done at all if you have spondylolisthesis (slipping of one vertebra over the other vertebra) or spinal stenosis (narrowing of the spinal canal in which the spinal cord travels). Back extension is another range of motion that is often measured at a physician's office, especially if he or she routinely treats back pain.

Side bending

Work on side bending to the left and then to the right. Remember to take a break and relax in between sides. You can accomplish this stretch by standing with feet shoulder-width apart, bending your right arm over your head, and holding your left arm by your side while reaching down to the ground as you bend to the left. Rest and relax. Do the same for the right side.

Rotational stretch

Place your hands on your hips. Standing straight with your feet shoulder-width apart, twist your torso, your left hip and your left arm (in unison) to the right. Rest and relax. Do the same for the right side.

Buttock Stretch

Lie flat on your back with your legs straight out. Bend the right knee. Lift the left leg and place the left ankle on top of the bent right knee. That might be enough of a stretch to start. If you do not feel anything, then reach behind your right knee with your hands and pull your right knee to your chest, using your arms. At this point, you might feel like you are a pretzel, and that is why some people call this the "pretzel stretch." Remember to hold the stretch for 30 seconds or as long as you can. Rest for a few seconds. Do the same for the other side.

Hamstring Stretch

Lie flat on your back with your legs straight out and shoulder-width apart. Bend the right knee. Lift the left leg straight up, trying to get it vertical to the ground. You may need a towel or a therapy band to lift your leg and feel a stretch in the left hamstring behind the upper part of the leg. Hold for 30 seconds or as long as you can, at least 5 seconds preferably. Rest. Do the same for the right side.

Pelvic Muscle Stretch

Lie down with arms at your sides and legs bent at the knees, shoulder-width apart, and your back against the floor. To start, make sure the small of your back is touching the floor. Try to push your back into the floor, pointing your pelvis to your chin. Take a break and do the opposite stretch, meaning pushing your pelvis toward your knees, which will lift the small of your back up off the floor, slightly.

Ankle Stretch

Lie flat on the ground with legs straight out. Point your right toes so that they push the sole of your foot to the ground. Another way of thinking about this motion is pointing your right toes away from your body. This motion flexes your ankle. Then, point your left toes so that they push the sole of your foot to the ground, pointing away from your body. Now, try to make your right toes touch your right shin (an impossible feat, but the idea gets the correct stretch). You could also think of it as pointing your right toes to the ceiling. After that, try to make your left toes touch your left shin, pointing them toward the ceiling.

Strengthening | The key to protecting your back

A strong back is your best weapon against further back injury and future exacerbations of your pain. Your core muscles are key to a strong back. The core muscles include those in your back, abdomen, buttock, and hips. Your arms and legs are important too, but your core is the key. An important and often-neglected muscle group is the group of muscles that are responsible for back extension.

You may be thinking that you have already tried physical therapy and strengthening without success. However, the big question is, Did you strengthen your back extensors? This is accomplished by doing Roman Chair exercises or other exercises on the floor where you lie on your stomach with your legs extended and lift your torso up while bending your back backward. Often these extension exercises are ignored, leaving the core imbalanced because most programs focus on the abdominal muscles. Both the front (abdominals) and the back (extensors) of the core need to be strong and in balance for a healthy back.

Your physician might prescribe physical therapy for you to get you started on strengthening exercises so that you are instructed in the proper way to perform each exercise. Depending on your individual needs, you might have two therapy sessions and then be transitioned to a home program. Alternatively, you might go through a four-week program and then be transitioned to a home program. Ideally, you will get to the point where you are performing strengthening exercises twice a week, independently, in your own home or in a gym.

Here are some examples of different exercises that your physician or therapist might recommend. As with stretching, it is important to strengthen opposing muscles, ones that cause flexion (forward bend) as well as ones that cause extension (backward bend) around a joint. Also similar to stretching, it is important to breathe as you perform these exercises. These exercises should not be painful. If you experience pain, stop and speak with your physician. Many of these exercises can be done while lying down. Variations of these exercises can be done with a therapeutic exercise ball or with resistance machines in a gym. Your physician or therapist will help you determine the best method for you. They will also tell you which exercises, if any, are contraindicated for you.

Back Extension Exercises

Lying on your stomach, with legs straight out and arms by your side, raise your head and torso off the floor. Breathe while holding the position for 5 seconds. Then, relax. Repeat 10 times.

Variation: Camel Stretch

Position yourself on your hands and knees with your neck parallel to the ground. Allow your back to sag into the ground such that your stomach pulls to the ground and your buttock pulls to the ceiling. Breathe and hold for 5 seconds. Then, relax. Repeat 10 times.

Abdominal Muscle Exercises (Flexion of Torso)

This exercise is known as the partial curl. It is performed lying on the floor with knees bent, shoulder-width apart, and arms straight down by your sides. Gently raise your head off the ground, tucking your chin to your chest. You can clasp your hands behind your head or hold your arms out straight by your sides. Next raise your head, shoulders, and upper back a few inches off the floor and hold for 5 seconds. Your hands can be behind your head in the raised position or they can be lifted off the ground, straight out by your sides. Relax and repeat 10 times.

Variation: Cat Stretch

Position yourself on your hands and knees with your neck parallel to the ground. Arch and round your back pushing it to the ceiling. Breathe and hold for 5 seconds. Then, relax. Repeat 10 times.

Hip Extensor Exercises

Lie down on your stomach with legs straight out and arms by your side. Lift the left leg with knee straight and raise it about 5 inches off the floor. Breathe and hold for 5 seconds. Relax and repeat 10 times. Then, alternate and do the same with the right leg.

Hip Flexor Exercises

Lie down on your back with legs straight out and arms by your side. Lift the left leg with knee straight and raise it about 5 inches off the floor. Breathe and hold for 5 seconds. Relax and repeat 10 times. Then, alternate and do the same with the right leg.

Back, Hip, and Leg Muscle Exercise

Stand up straight with your back against a wall and arms down by your side. Slowly and gently slide down the wall by bending your knees, keeping your back up against the wall. Continue to slide down until you are in a sitting position creating a 90-degree angle between your waist and legs. Breathe and hold for 5 seconds. Then, slowly slide your way back up the wall to a standing position while breathing. Relax and repeat 10 times.

These are just a few examples of the possible exercises that you can do to help strengthen your back. Your physician or therapist will have more specific suggestions that will suit your unique needs.

After performing strengthening exercises, you might feel some soreness in the areas that you worked. This is normal and to be expected. People with back pain and people without back pain can experience this same soreness. Basically, it is a sign that your muscles are working and changes are happening inside the muscles. The soreness only lasts two to three days. Thus, strengthening exercises are recommended twice a week. Often anti-inflammatory medications can help relieve the soreness. Before taking any over-the-counter medications, however, you should speak to your physician, because they might be contraindicated for you, or they may interfere with your current medications.

There are some useful Web sites that offer videos of stretches and strengthening exercises. You might find these helpful to view before you get started. Here are some suggested sites:

- The National Library of Medicine
  www.nlm.nih.gov/medlineplus/backpain.html
- Mayo Clinic
  www.mayoclinic.com/health/back-pain
- American Academy of Orthopedic Surgeons
  www.orthoinfo.aaos.org
- University of Michigan Medical Center
  www.med.umich.edu/1libr/guides/adult%20LBP%20Exercise.pdf

Exercise Your Way to a Healthy Back | Start today

Starting an exercise program involves more than merely deciding to do it. It takes a realistic consideration of lifestyle and circumstances and a commitment to devote the necessary time and energy. First, you have to set aside time for exercise. Most good regimens require at least 15 to 30 minutes a day. Then, you need to consider where you will exercise. Perform your exercises on a firm but comfortable surface, such as carpet or an exercise mat. Never exercise on a bed or couch, as these surfaces are too soft and won't support the low back. And, finally, there is the need to start slowly and progress at your own pace so that you don't run into problems at the outset. It's okay to start with only a few repetitions that pose minimal challenge. As you begin, don't be intimidated by small aches and mild muscle fatigue, especially if you haven't stretched your back for a while. As you get stronger and your endurance improves, increase the number of repetitions.

Remember not to undertake exercise without talking to your physician. This is especially true if you are experiencing numbness in the genital area; loss of bowel, bladder, or sexual functioning; or muscle weakness in the lower extremities. Don't set yourself up for failure by starting an exercise program in the midst of an acute pain attack. Wait until it passes.

Tell family and friends that you've started an exercise program. A public statement makes the effort more concrete, and their support will keep you going when you feel like you're failing. It's also helpful to get an "exercise buddy," someone who shares your commitment and desire to exercise and stay motivated throughout the process.

Beyond Stretching and Strengthening

Once you have become more physically active by incorporating lifestyle exercise as well as stretching and strengthening into your daily routine, you may want to consider adding other types of exercise, preferably a physical activity that is safe and one that you truly enjoy. If you like an activity, then you are more likely to stick with it. Don't pick something that you think you *should* do. Pick something that you *want* to do.

There are certain activities that do not mix well with back pain, such as water skiing, sledding, ice hockey, football, soccer, volleyball, weight lifting, and jumping on a trampoline. The sudden jarring motion, the sudden twisting and turning, and the physical contact involved in these sports make them poor and even dangerous choices for back pain patients. Although it is not likely that many of you were considering joining a football team or going water skiing, knowing these parameters and general guidelines may be helpful to you.

Think back to your youth and recall physical activities that you enjoyed. Perhaps you can still do that activity or perhaps you can make modifications to it. Some popular choices for people with back pain include walking, bicycling on a stationary bike, yoga, and water activities. We will discuss the last two activities in more detail.

Yoga

Yoga is based on the premise that physical, mental, and spiritual energy are intertwined and can enhance overall health and well-being. Yogic theory holds that our minds are agitated and restless, which leads to anxiety. This anxiety in turn negatively impacts the health of our bodies, leading to disease and decreased mental strength.

Yoga is much more than a few floor exercises. It is a holistic approach that utilizes both physical and psychological practices in an effort to decrease mental, emotional, and physical stress. To take full advantage of this Eastern method, yoga should be done initially with a trained instructor. Hatha yoga is probably the most common type of yoga for improving low back pain.

Yoga in general is based on the three principles of asana (posture), pranayama (breathing), and samadhi (meditation). During the poses, or asanas, an immobile bodily posture is maintained in an attempt to isolate the mind by freeing it from attention to bodily functions. Pranayama focuses on regulating breathing, which in yoga is thought to be "the life force." Pranayama exercises promote the proper flow of life force throughout the body so that a rhythmic state of relaxation can take place. This prepares the body for the next step: meditation. Samadhi, or spiritual realization, is the accumulation of disciplined practice. When patients achieve this state of relaxation and meditation, the result is reduced muscle tension, slower heart rate, lower blood pressure, decreased brain wave patterns, improved immune function, and decreased pain.

Yoga can be highly effective for low back pain because it can help improve posture, increase strength and flexibility, and provide an overall state of relaxation. When first learning yoga, seek out a qualified yoga instructor who listens to your concerns and takes your problems into consideration in devising a yoga plan for you. For example, several positions can be modified to accommodate back problems. Everyone and every back problem is different, so you need to listen to your body and not risk re-injury.

Water Activities

Water activities are an excellent form of exercise for people with chronic low back pain. Water makes us buoyant, so the joints experience less pressure and stress. Water therapy is a great way to start. It can provide relief from pain because there is little resistance to body movements. Just as physical therapy can be active or passive, so can water therapy.

With active therapy, you are proactively doing something, like coordinating exercises that target your problem areas. Passive therapy includes sitting in a hot tub or whirlpool where the motion and heat of the water soothes painful muscles but doesn't assist in the healing process. Passive therapy is best used initially during a flare-up. Then, as the pain level returns to baseline, proceed with a water therapy program that will strengthen muscles and reduce pain.

There are many different activities to enjoy in the water. Many people like walking in water better than walking on dry land. You can walk laps in the shallow end of a pool from one side to the other. There are also water aerobic classes. Swimming is an activity that is easy on the joints and one that works many different muscle groups. You might call the local YMCA and ask about their programs. Many rehabilitation facilities also have pools. Speak to your physician and find out if water activities might be right for you.

Road Map for Getting Moving | Ten basic steps

1. Make an appointment with your physician and discuss physical activity. Your doctor may advise you to begin with physical or occupational therapy.
2. Select a physical activity you enjoy. Be creative. Make modifications, if necessary. Spend time on the selection process and be willing to change activities to prevent boredom. Cross training, doing more than one type of physical activity during the week, is a good idea to keep you engaged.
3. Set a day and time to begin. Mark it on a calendar, and just do it.
4. Share your plans and your progress with people who care about you. If you can enlist a friend to join you, great.
5. Start low and go slow. You might begin by walking around the

inside of your house, walking around your block, walking around a track, or walking around a mall. Exercise a little longer each week. Initially, don't shoot for the moon. Reach for a streetlight, and enjoy the feeling of success. Success breeds success.

6. Make physical activity a part of your daily routine. Keep a chart of your efforts and make sure to share your progress with your physician.

7. Aim to stretch three to five times a week, strengthen your muscles twice a week, and do aerobic activity five days a week.

8. Some is better than none. If one week you can only manage to be physically active three out of five days, be positive and realize that three days is better than two days. Two days are better than one day, and, of course, one day is better than none.

9. Set realistic goals for yourself each week. Write them down to keep yourself accountable. Mark them in your calendar, as if they were important appointments you need to keep, because they are.

10. Celebrate your efforts. When you meet your goals, reward yourself with healthy prizes, such as a massage or trip to a spa. You may become so active that you need new sneakers or athletic attire. It is important to take the time to feel good about your efforts and yourself.

After reading this chapter, we hope you feel like moving around. In fact, if you are so inclined, place a bookmark in the book and stand up and stretch. Hold the stretch for 30 seconds while continuing to breathe comfortably. Perhaps go for a walk around the block or around your kitchen table. Experience what it feels like to be active. Think about the changes that occur in your muscle cells and in your brain cells when you become physically active. Remember the best ways to protect your back are to strengthen your core muscles, increase your flexibility, and be physically active on a daily basis. You can do it.

Chapter 6
Tools for Reducing Stress

Positive thoughts lead to positive results.

THE MANY FACTORS THAT influence back pain include the physical, as found in pain flares; the emotional, as expressed in anger or sadness; and the mental, as exhibited in depression or negative self-talk. The mind and body are not separate entities; rather, they are interconnected and dependent upon each another for harmony. How you feel, whether happy, sad, angry, or frustrated, will have a direct impact on your pain state. Perhaps you have experienced what some patients report: that their pain is significantly less when their mind is occupied with watching television or reading a book. This is an example of how the mind-body connection can be used to change the perception of pain. Consider the possibilities.

Decrease Stress | Reduce pain

Pain and stress go hand in hand, and when you experience pain you are less able to deal with the everyday stressors that are a normal part of living. Stress intensifies feelings of anger, sadness, and worthlessness. It can also increase pain levels as you tighten muscles and create muscle fatigue and strain. Pain causes stress, which in turn intensifies pain.

Think about the last stressful event you encountered. Do you remember how it felt? Your heart rate probably quickened and your skin felt cool to the touch. You may have broken out in a sweat. Physically you react to a stressful event by releasing hormones that cause your body to go into hyper drive. This is called the fight-or-flight phenomenon.

Stress can be positive or negative. Positive stress provides the typical feelings of excitement and happiness, as with a job change or the arrival of a new addition to the family. Negative stress can include financial difficulties, marital discord, or chronic pain. With these stressors you feel out of sorts and have difficulty concentrating. Prolonged negative stress not only intensifies the chronic pain state but can also have a detrimental effect on your overall health. Negative stress weakens the immune system, leaving your body vulnerable to illness, and can strain the cardiovascular system, leading to serious complications. Stress triggers can occur without our awareness, so identifying them is essential to eliminating them. Some triggers may be external, like family, work, or the environment. Other triggers may be internal, like poor health habits or the pressures of perfectionism. Start by identifying your triggers. Make a note each time you feel stressed; record the circumstances surrounding that occurrence; figure out what you can do to reduce your exposure; and focus on the things you can control. Because completely avoiding all sources of stress is unrealistic, incorporating stress busters into your daily routine is essential for improving the quality of your life.

Look at your list: What have you identified as triggers for stress? Are you trying to accomplish too much too quickly? Are you expecting yourself to be organized when you're generally not? When you have identified your unreasonable expectations, consider making basic changes to your routine.

There are many alterations you can make. For example, simplify your schedule and pace yourself. What can you eliminate? What can you delegate? Stop accepting additional responsibilities. Tell yourself that it's okay to say "no," thereby bestowing upon yourself a sense of empowerment. Plan your day the evening beforehand, and wake up 15 minutes early so you don't feel rushed and stressed.

Remember to take breaks, eat well, get enough sleep, and think good thoughts. Go for a walk or stretch periodically throughout the day. Maintain a diet rich in fruits and vegetables, because the body requires a variety of nutrients to stay healthy. Get enough sleep to allow your brain to file the new information you acquire each day and for your body to reenergize itself for the next day. Try to keep a consistent sleep schedule. Most of all, remain positive. Avoid self-deprecating talk and replace it with positive reinforcement.

Relax | Give yourself a break

Extensive research has been done on the positive effects of relaxation. Performing relaxation techniques can have an immediate impact, by lowering heart rate, breathing rate, and blood pressure. In the long term, taking time out has been shown to decrease stress and pain. Relaxation techniques are a natural part of our lives. We often take them for granted, however, and therefore sometimes overlook the fact that they are always available for our benefit. Some effective relaxation techniques are deep breathing, word repetition, guided imagery, and progressive muscle relaxation.

Deep breathing can decrease stress when practiced in a slow and methodical way. Individuals who breathe from the chest have greater tension and stress in their neck and shoulders. In deep breathing, you inhale not from the chest, which is shallow, but from the diaphragm, which yields more complete expansion. It also allows for a greater exchange of carbon dioxide, which in turn gives you additional energy. Ultimately, diaphragmatic breathing can be combined with other relaxation techniques.

To assess how you breathe, place one hand on your chest and the other on your stomach, close your eyes, and concentrate. If your chest moves up and down in response to your breathing, you are likely a chest breather and you need to learn how to use your abdominal muscles to breathe differently. Now, try to take a series of deep breaths—in your nose and out your mouth. Do you feel that sense of relaxation? Incorporating a few minutes of diaphragmatic breathing throughout the day is one way to decrease your stress. Deliberate breathing, as with any relaxation technique, takes time to master. Start with a few minutes each day and try to work up to a session of 15 to 20 minutes daily.

Word repetition, or cue-controlled relaxation, involves choosing a word or series of words that is soothing to you and repeating it whenever you feel stressed. The purpose is to refocus your mind away from the stress or pain. Take, for example, the words "I am calm." As you slowly say them, inhale deeply. As you say the last word, slowly exhale. Repeating the words over and over again while at the same time breathing deeply will give you a sense of calm.

Guided imagery is the technique of picturing yourself in a place that is peaceful. It might be a sandy beach in the middle of nowhere or it might be a hammock under a sunny blue sky. The key to guided imagery is to engage your sensory memory: feel the warm sun on your skin, hear the waves of the ocean, and picture the colors of the sky. The message sent to your brain by these images is what produces the relaxation. Imagery can decrease your perception of pain by temporarily removing you from the pain state.

Many people also use guided imagery to enhance their physical healing, notably people with cancer who visualize their chemotherapy attacking the affected area. People dealing with chronic low back pain can utilize this same technique. Imagine a large knot in your back and then focus on gradually opening that knot, with the loosening representing decreased muscle tension. Imagery has been shown to provide a calming distraction for people undergoing medical procedures. While you're focusing on that sandy beach and the feeling of sand between your toes, you are distracted from feeling your pain.

Progressive muscle relaxation involves tensing and relaxing a particular muscle group, one at a time. People who find it difficult to relax by sitting quietly may find this activity helpful. Progressive muscle relaxation works when you contract the muscles in a body part and then release the tension by slowly relaxing those muscles. For example, start by tensing and relaxing your shoulder muscles. Then move on to your arm muscles, the muscles in your hands and fingers, your chest muscles, stomach muscles, and so on. When utilizing this technique, you are learning to tell the difference between tense and relaxed states, and you are developing your skills of observation.

Relaxation won't eliminate your pain, but it will reduce your anxiety and give you a greater sense of control. Chronic pain leads to chronic stress, which disrupts the natural balance our bodies rely upon for well-being. Relaxation techniques will help restore balance to your life and ultimately diminish your pain state. Regular practice will also help you recognize the difference between sore, tense muscles and relaxed, comfortable ones. When done consistently, relaxation will help you deal with the physical and emotional demands of your daily life with greater ease.

Like any method, relaxation takes time to learn. You may not notice an immediate benefit, but continue doing whichever technique is most comfortable for you until relaxation becomes second nature. Wear comfortable clothing that makes it easy to move around, and be patient with yourself—these techniques are meant to decrease your stress, not add to it.

Biofeedback | Control your body's responses

Biofeedback is a form of intensive training designed to consciously influence a physical response. Its purpose is to cultivate the person's ability to control his or her body's reaction to a particular stimulus. For example, if you are experiencing a muscle spasm that is making your low back pain worse, then a key to reducing your discomfort could be learning ways to control the spasm.

Biofeedback training is a painless, noninvasive procedure that involves placing electrodes on the skin in an effort to monitor the muscle that is tense and needs retraining. It's called electromyography or EMG biofeedback. A computer is connected to the electrodes and the computer reads the amount of electrical activity related to the level of rigidity in the muscle. You view the amount of muscle tension on a computer monitor and start to learn new ways to decrease the tightness. Your brain will assist in the retraining method because it sees what the muscle looks like when it is stressed and when it is relaxed.

Respiration feedback is another type of biofeedback. The rate, rhythm, and volume of each breath is measured to help you incorporate diaphragmatic breathing into your care plan.

Most specialists in biofeedback recommend a short trial of five to fifteen sessions. Biofeedback can be useful not only for retraining tense muscles but for also controlling the anxiety that accompanies chronic pain. As with many other approaches to retraining the mind, there are few scientific studies regarding the long-term effectiveness of biofeedback. However, biofeedback is considered mainstream therapy, not a complementary and alternative medicine (CAM), and therefore it is reimbursable by many insurance companies. There are multiple studies on the effectiveness of biofeedback, including several Cochrane Reviews[1]—summaries produced by a group of health care experts who analyze all of the literature on a particular topic, separate the good from the bad studies, and render an opinion. Although it has been found that biofeedback does not work for everyone, many people who have used it and believe in it in principle have shown an overall reduction in pain levels.

Hypnosis | Concentrate

Hypnosis is a natural state of intense concentration that can be used to achieve total and complete relaxation. What constitutes hypnosis is the subject of much debate among experts in the field. Hypnosis relies on control of the body and the mind. Hypnosis evolved from techniques explored by Franz Anton Mesmer more than 200 years ago and is used today to treat a host of conditions from anxiety and stress to chronic pain conditions. It can also be used to help people lose weight and stop smoking. Like biofeedback, hypnosis is considered mainstream and not a complementary and alternative medicine. It is reimbursable by many insurance companies and is well researched. A licensed health care provider, such as a physician or psychologist, can introduce you to the benefits of hypnosis. In time, you may be able to successfully achieve self-hypnosis.

The hypnotic induction process involves three parts: relaxation, imagery, and suggestion.

Relaxation is typically achieved by taking several slow, deep breaths, allowing a good feeling to overcome your body. You let your muscles and limbs grow limp.

Imagery, which is next, is used to deepen the level of relaxation. You may be told to picture someone walking down a flight of stairs, while counting backwards from ten. With each number, you descend one stair and with each stair you relax further. Picture a feather bed at the base of the stairs, and when you get to the bottom of the stairs, picture yourself sinking into that bed and resting your head on a deep soft pillow.

Suggestion, the third part of hypnosis, is used to bring about a change in your subconscious. Your brain has both a conscious level and a subconscious level. Operating on the theory that if you *think* you have less pain you will *feel* less pain, you work on making your brain believe it. In your deeply relaxed state, this suggestion to your subconscious brain can work. For some people the suggestion takes hold immediately; for others, it is necessary to repeat the suggestion over several days or even for a couple of weeks to get it to take up residence in the subconscious, helping to reduce the pain state. Although hypnosis cannot alter something that is unchangeable, such as restore your vision if you are blind, it can help in a variety of changeable behaviors, such as sleep patterns or eating habits or pain patterns.

Several misconceptions exist about hypnosis, including the belief that it induces a state of deep sleep. Hypnosis is actually a state of complete relaxation in which you are still able to hear, speak, and move around. You cannot be hypnotized against your will, nor can you be forced to do anything you wouldn't normally do. Common roadblocks to becoming hypnotized include trying too hard, fear, misconceptions about hypnosis, and an unconscious desire to hold on to the pain state.

Currently there are no reported stories of injury involving the use of hypnosis; however, the World Health Organization does not recommend the use of hypnosis on people with a history of psychosis or other specific psychiatric conditions.

Music Therapy | Listen to soothing sounds

Music can excite us and make us want to sing and dance with joy; it can ignite our feelings of patriotism, summon memories from the past, and engage our emotions. Music can also relax us, and it is this kind of music that can soothe a person with pain. Research has shown that appropriate music can have a positive effect on heart rate and blood pressure. Environmental sounds such as falling rain or rolling ocean waves help some people. Find the music or sound that soothes you best and listen to it often.

The Multipronged Approach | Seek the help of professionals

If your doctor recommends a psychologist or psychiatrist as part of a multipronged approach, you may say to yourself, "Hey I'm not crazy! I really do hurt." You need to know that your doctor does not doubt the reality of your pain; rather, he or she is acknowledging that certain emotions, like depression and anxiety, can magnify your pain, making it worse than it needs to be.

The discomfort that you're experiencing affects not only your body but your mind as well. Using a psychologist or psychiatrist is another way to help you deal with your circumstances. Maybe you've already tried medication and physical therapy; just think of this approach as physical therapy for your mind. Psychology and psychiatry are different specialties, and sometimes you might work with a person in each field.

A *psychologist* is a professional trained in the area of mental disorders, emotions, and behaviors. Licensed psychologists have earned a doctorate in psychology and are qualified to work with you through one-on-one sessions or in a group setting. They listen to you very carefully and they offer guidance and suggestions (this interaction is often called "talk therapy"). They are not medical doctors and therefore cannot prescribe medication. Not all psychologists are trained to help patients deal with pain; helping people in pain requires specialized knowledge.

A *psychiatrist* is a medical doctor who pursued a residency in the area of psychiatry. Psychiatrists discuss the problem with the patient and often prescribe medication. Psychiatrists often also work with psychologists, who may undertake more intensive talk therapy than psychiatrists, in an effort to help patients achieve their goals—in this case, pain management.

Social workers may also be helpful. Many of them have specialized training and education in treating people with chronic pain. Social workers can also help with other concerns, such as finances and vocational rehabilitation.

Some patients have found that one-on-one counseling with their pastor or spiritual leader is helpful. While this can be beneficial initially, I recommend seeking a licensed professional who has the additional training and education to deal with chronic pain patients.

When you are in a chronic pain state, your life is typically all about your condition. Chronic pain is disruptive; consequently, anxiety and depression may set in early on. If anxiety and depression are not treated, pain symptoms may become worse and more difficult to control. Anxiety often stems from a fear of additional suffering, so addressing your mental and emotional health must be part of your approach to pain management. Symptoms of depression include increased pain, a greater need for sleep, thoughts of sadness and hopelessness, and a decreased desire to do the activities you usually enjoy.

If you have any thoughts of suicide, they need to be addressed immediately. Please seek out a friend, family member, religious leader, or your doctor if you are experiencing any thoughts of suicide. You or they may want to call 1-800-suicide or go to the Web site www.suicide.com.

It is my strong recommendation that if you are having suicidal thoughts without having immediate intentions, you should contact your doctor right away. If suicidal thoughts dominate your thinking and you have considered how you might kill yourself, you should go to the emergency room. Family members may have no idea how to deal with someone who is having thoughts of suicide. The focus of this book is to gain the skills to take back control of your life. Suicide is never the answer.

Though I will discuss various medicines, including antidepressants, in the next chapter, it is not enough to simply get a prescription for an antidepressant. You need to analyze what is at the root of your depression and anxiety and look for ways to minimize the cause. Just as negative self-talk can have a detrimental effect on controlling pain, so can a defeated frame of mind. Working with a psychologist or psychiatrist can help you identify ways to better control pain by reexamining your thoughts and feelings. Being open to a wide range of healing modalities is the best way to overcome pain.

Chapter 7
Pain Medications

Medications can control symptoms and help give you a better quality of life.

Of the many tools available for managing pain, one of the most effective is prescription medicine. This chapter provides an overview of some of the best medications available in the market today. Although you may find this chapter somewhat technical when it is describing medicines you don't take, you will probably find it interesting when it addresses the medications you have heard of, are presently taking, or have taken in the past. You can see where your medication or medications fit into the larger picture. As with all therapies, you and your doctor must evaluate the various options and decide which medications might best help you.

There are many factors to consider when choosing pain medication, among them:

- Is your pain acute or chronic?
- Has it just started, or have you had the pain for a long time?
- Will your insurance plan cover the cost of the medication?
- Do you have other financial resources to help pay for medication?
- Do you have a support system that can help you? How large and reliable is it?
- Will you be able to follow dosing instructions and take medicine properly?

In an ideal world, you would be able to pursue every avenue for relief, but in reality, insurance coverage may approve only some of the treatments and even then only particular applications for a specified period of time. Unfortunately, the more limited your financial resources are, the more limited your treatment options will be. A strong support system made up of your family and friends can provide you with valuable assistance in coping with pain.

Prescription medication is a valuable tool that every physician can use in treating his or her patients' pain. Medicines can be prescribed to treat the actual pain or one of several disorders that go along with pain—such as depression, insomnia, and anxiety. There are a variety of options to choose from, including:

analgesics,
antidepressants,
antiepileptics,
muscle relaxants,
sodium and calcium channel antagonists, and
topicals (medications applied to the skin).

Medications can reduce the perception of pain. When combined with restored function they can improve a person's quality of life. With proper medications you may be able to perform regular activities around the house, find work possible instead of unbearable, and improve your relationships.

Pharmaceutical companies provide guides for the proper doses of their medications, but the best dose for each patient still may not be clear. For pain medications of all types, physicians often must individualize dosing schedules for each patient. That's why doctors often increase the medication incrementally, step by step, to reach the point of optimal benefit and fewest possible side effects.

Pharmaceutical companies also provide cautions relating to possible drug interactions along with complete descriptions of each medication to help patients better understand the medicine they are taking. Some medications interact with other medications in a way that can make them either less or more effective—or even dangerous. To avoid adverse drug interactions, let your physician know all the medications, prescribed and otherwise, that you take. Different disease states can also affect the way the body responds to medications, which is why your physician should be aware of all your illnesses—not only your low back pain.

Doctors tend to start with the medications that can give the most benefit with the fewest side effects. Doses are increased as tolerated. Patients who take an active role in the use of their medications have the best success. I recommend that you keep a list of all of the medications you use, including the dosage and frequency, and bring this to the appointments with your health care provider. Know why you are using a medication. Tune in to the effects of the medication so you are able to tell your doctor how it helps, or doesn't, and about any corresponding side effects. Read, commit to memory, and file all the medication information given to you by your doctor or pharmacist. Consider using a loose-leaf binder to organize this information. In addition to keeping the fact sheets you can include blank pages on which to record your responses to your medications.

Take your medications as you and your physician agree you will; if you want to change the way you are using a medicine, contact your physician first. Continually reassess the effects of your medications. What helps today may not help tomorrow. Your body can develop tolerances to the medications, or different disease states can develop while you are using a medicine. Some people do well by keeping a daily diary describing the status of their disease and the effects of the medications (see chapter 4 for one example of a diary format).

Analgesics | Pain-relieving medications

Medications that relieve pain are called analgesics. There are three classifications of analgesics: nonsteroidals, also known as NSAIDs; tramadol-related products; and opioids.

The term *analgesic drug* can be somewhat ambiguous. Drugs can have multiple uses, and it is often the use that really determines whether we are thinking of the drug as an analgesic or not. For example, while hydrocodone, found in common medications such as Lortab and Vicodin, is a good analgesic, it is also commonly used as an antitussive or cough medicine. So, in one setting hydrocodone is an analgesic while in another setting it is a cough medication. More recently some antidepressants, such as Cymbalta, and antiepileptics, such as Lyrica, have been classified as analgesics and approved by the Food and Drug Administration (FDA) for labeling as pain relievers for certain types of nerve injury–related pain.

Traditional analgesic medications—NSAIDs, tramadol, and opioids —interrupt the pain signal by acting at several different sites in the pain-processing pathway. Generally, as one proceeds from nonsteroidals to tramadol and opioids, the strength of the medication increases. Guidelines provided by the World Health Organization recommend starting with the weakest analgesic and progressing to the strongest as needed, but the health care professional is free to use discretion in deciding where along the analgesic continuum a patient should start. All classes of analgesics can cause side effects, some of them quite noticeable.

Nonsteroidals (NSAIDs)

The first class of analgesic pain relievers to consider are the nonsteroidals, a diverse group of medications that alter the pain perception by changing the production of prostaglandins in the body. Prostaglandins are chemicals that can be released from cells and cause pain in certain settings. The result is varying degrees of pain relief as well as a reduction in inflammation and temperature. In the list below, some commonly used prescription nonsteroidals are shown with the generic name of the drug first and brand name(s) shown in parentheses:

aspirin
celecoxib (Celebrex)
choline magnesium trisalicylate
   (Trilisate)
diclofenac and misoprostol
   (Arthrotec—a pill combining
   Voltaren and Cytotec)
diclofenac potassium (Cataflam)
diclofenac sodium (Voltaren)
diflunisal (Dolobid)
etodolac (Lodine)
fenoprofen (Nalfon)
flurbiprofen (Ansaid)
ibuprofen (Advil, Motrin)

indomethacin (Indocin)
ketoprofen (Actron, Orudis)
ketorolac (Toradol)
meclofenamate (Meclofen)
mefenamic acid (Ponstel)
meloxicam (Mobic)
nabumetone (Relafen)
naproxen (Anaprox, Naprelan,
   Naprosyn, among others)
oxaprozin (Daypro)
piroxicam (Feldene)
salsalate (Disalcid)
sulindac (Clinoril)
tolmetin (Tolectin)

These medications are usually the first analgesics a doctor considers, because when used with opioids, they can reduce the amount of opioid needed to provide pain relief. This approach is known as opioid sparing. In addition, nonsteroidals can act synergistically with opioids; that is, the effect of using them together is greater than what can be achieved by either alone. But there is a ceiling effect with nonsteroidal medications. Beyond a certain dose, no greater benefit will be obtained.

Complications of NSAIDs

Though commonly used, these medications can potentially cause problems with many organ systems. One study showed the greatest risk for developing a stomach ulcer is with indomethacin, tolmetin, and meclofenamate; the least with aspirin, salsalate, and ibuprofen. The most common problems with these medications include stomach aches, ulcers, and bleeding. If severe bleeding occurs, it can be life threatening. Unfortunately, if these medications are harming your stomach, there may be no symptoms to warn you of the problem. Within one week of starting nonsteroidals, one out of three patients shows changes in the lining of the stomach. Hundreds of thousands of people subsequently seek medical care for nonsteroidal-induced stomach damage, and these side effects tend to increase with age. The longer you take a nonsteroidal, the higher the likelihood that you will develop a complication. Factors that increase your risk of having stomach problems include: age, prior stomach problems, steroid use, alcohol use, and the use of more than one NSAID at a time. But many stomach problems can be limited or prevented with the concurrent use of misoprostol (Cytotec), omeprazole (Prilosec), or similar types of medications.

Almost one out of five people using nonsteroidals will experience a decrease in kidney function. This decrease is most significant in individuals over the age of 65 and individuals with a medical history of heart failure, renal insufficiency, and hepatic insufficiency. Some will show changes in their kidney function within three days of beginning a medication regimen. Unchecked kidney dysfunction can lead to kidney failure, the need for dialysis, and even death. In addition, because NSAIDs inhibit the production of prostaglandins in the kidney, patients may retain fluids and experience a higher blood pressure.

NSAIDs are metabolized by the liver. They must be used with caution in people who have any liver dysfunction. In extremely rare cases, NSAIDs have caused liver damage leading to death.

All NSAIDs affect the cardiovascular system and its function to varying degrees. With the exceptions of Celebrex, Disalcid, and Trilisate, all NSAIDs inhibit platelet aggregation. They interact with warfarin (Coumadin), so the dose of Coumadin usually must be reduced. All NSAIDs are now known to affect the chance of having a cardiovascular event; you may be more likely to have a heart attack while taking an NSAID than if you were not taking the medication. If you have a history of congestive heart failure, you are twice as likely to be hospitalized when starting an NSAID than if you were on a different medication. This increased risk should be discussed with your doctor before starting and continuing your NSAID; the benefits need to outweigh the risks.

Since NSAIDs can also predispose people to develop bleeding ulcers, the use of a platelet inhibitor along with another anticoagulant can increase the risk of serious bleeding should an ulcer occur. The effect on bleeding is somewhat complicated because certain NSAIDs, such as aspirin, interfere with platelet function and can cause increased bleeding, often seen as easy bruising in patients prescribed aspirin after a heart attack or stroke. Other NSAIDs, such as Bextra and Vioxx, have been found to cause increased blood clotting and a heightened risk of heart attack and have therefore been pulled from the market. To further complicate matters, the NSAIDs Celebrex, Disalcid, and Trilisate do not change platelet function in any noticeable fashion. Although it is beyond the scope of this book to explain in depth why different NSAIDs have different effects on platelet function, you can understand some of the challenges that physician and patient face when developing a medication regimen. Many factors influence the choice of an NSAID for a particular patient.

Owing to the potential problems that can occur with nonsteroidals, new, apparently safer, classes of medications have been developed over the last several years, and celecoxib (Celebrex) is the best example. Celebrex helps reduce pain and inflammation with fewer corresponding problems in the stomach and no effect on platelets. Currently, it appears that the cardiovascular risk from Celebrex is no greater than that of any of the older NSAIDs. Given that the use of Celebrex carries less risk of stomach damage or bleeding from interference with platelet function, it is often considered the best NSAID for long-term use. As with all NSAIDs, however, there is still a risk of fluid retention and kidney damage.

When Celebrex cannot be used, Mobic (meloxicam) and Arthrotec should be considered next. Mobic is reputed to cause fewer stomach problems than the other nonsteroidals. Arthrotec has a nonsteroidal agent (diclofenac, whose brand name is Voltaren) combined with an agent (misoprostol, brand name Cytotec) to protect the stomach.

Acetaminophen (Tylenol) is not technically considered an NSAID. It has no peripheral anti-inflammatory effect. But it is a popular alternative to NSAIDs due to its lack of effect on platelets, stomach, bone, and kidney. It has the potential to harm the liver, however, if not used as directed. Indeed, at one time acetaminophen was a leading cause of death from drug overdose. Despite these facts, acetaminophen when used in recommended doses remains a very useful drug for everyday aches and pains.

Tramadol

Generally stronger than aspirin but weaker than pure opioids, tramadol, which has been available in the United States for more than ten years in the form of Ultram and Ultracet, is the next step in pain relief. An extended release form of tramadol, Ultram ER, has recently entered the marketplace. Tramadol is a codeine analog and has fewer side effects than the NSAIDs. (An analog is an agent with a chemical structure similar to the original medication, with corresponding comparable chemical effects—like siblings who behave in the same way.) Tramadol acts primarily by increasing serotonin and norepinephrine in the central nervous system. In addition, tramadol binds weakly to opioid receptors and has not been deemed a controlled substance by the Drug Enforcement Agency (DEA). Yet it is thought to be 20 percent as strong as morphine, with label indications recommending it for moderate to severe pain.

Seven percent of Caucasians cannot metabolize tramadol and therefore will not respond to its pain-relieving effects. The pain benefit peaks 2 hours after the initial dose and lasts approximately 6 hours. It can increase the drowsiness effects of a sedating agent when the two are used at the same time. Though generally well tolerated, tramadol can elicit side effects that may prompt discontinuation of use, including dizziness, lethargy, nausea, vomiting, and constipation. Many of these side effects will decrease over time with continued use of the drug. Increasing the dose slowly over time may improve tolerance.

This medication is a first choice agent for pain relief for people who cannot use nonsteroidals and opioids. It has been shown to be effective in patient groups experiencing chronic low back pain. Dosing varies, usually from one to eight pills per day. More than eight daily doses are discouraged because that amount would lower the seizure threshold and might induce a serotonin syndrome, which is a potentially life-threatening adverse drug reaction. Tramadol can also be found in mixture drugs, such as Ultracet and Ultram ER. Ultracet has 37.5 mg of tramadol combined with 325 mg of acetaminophen in each pill. A person can use up to ten pills per day and still stay below the daily maximum recommended dosages of tramadol and acetaminophen. I would not recommend this medication for any individual with a history of seizures/epilepsy, head trauma, alcohol or drug withdrawal, or any other known trauma to the central nervous system, because these problems could be made worse by this medication. Elderly people as well as people with known liver and kidney disease should take lower doses.

Opioids

The strongest class of pain-relieving medications are opioids. Opioids occur endogenously (naturally in the body) and exogenously (grown or synthesized outside the body). They modulate pain signals being transferred in the nervous system. They strongly affect the emotional component of pain.

Opioids are legally controlled substances. Their potential to create dependence, addiction, tolerance, and pseudoaddiction must be taken into account when considering these medications for pain control. Only when the first two levels of pain relievers have not yielded satisfactory results or when their risks outweigh their benefits will a physician turn to opioids for his or her patient. Opioids primarily work by binding to receptors in cell membranes in the central nervous system. The binding changes a cell's function; the net total result is that pain signals are altered, pupils constricted, emotions enhanced, and bowels slowed.

A wide range of options exists in this class of medication. The DEA has graded and regulated opioids, with classes II through IV relevant to managing back pain. The higher the numbered class, the less assumed risk of addiction. (We say "assumed" here because while the degree of risk has not been proven, it is generally believed to be in the range indicated by the numbered class system). Classes III and IV include mixed opioids such as codeine with Tylenol or aspirin. Class III agents include mixed agonist-antagonists, such as Suboxone or Talwin; these agents can give pain relief but, unlike pure agonist opioids, they have a ceiling for an analgesic effect—in other words, these agents come to a peak after which no additional benefits will be obtained. Class II opioids have the highest risk of addiction and are among the most potent agents at the physician's disposal. Common opioids include the following:

Class IV
propoxyphene (Darvon, Darvocet)

Class III
buprenorphine and naloxone (Suboxone)
codeine (Tylenol No. 2 to No. 4)
hydrocodone (Lorcet, Lortab, Norco, Vicodin)
pentazocine (Talwin)

Class II
codeine
fentanyl (Actiq, Duragesic, Fentora, Onsalis)
hydromorphone (Dilaudid)
meperidine (Demerol)
methadone (Dolophine)
morphine (Avinza, Embeda, Kadian, MS Contin, Oramorph)
oxycodone (OxyContin, Percocet, Percodan)
oxymorphone (Opana)
tapentadol (Nucynta)

Opioids can be administered by a number of methods:

- orally (by mouth)
  - as a pill or a liquid that is swallowed
  - through the lining of tissue in the mouth as a rapidly dissolving tablet either through the cheek tissue inside the mouth (buccal) or under the tongue (sublingual)
- rectally (as a suppository)

- inserted through a stoma (a surgically created opening on the abdomen that leads to the intestines) or any other opening in the body with mucosa
- subcutaneously (injected into a muscle or under the skin)
- intravenously (through a needle into a vein)
- epidurally (injected into the spinal cord)
- intrathecally (injected into the fluid around the spinal cord)
- transdermally (through a patch worn on the skin)

The oral route—liquids or pills that are swallowed—is the method recommended by many pain management experts because medication by mouth is both easy to use and easy to adjust dosages for.

Narcotics that can give pain relief for 8 or more hours are called sustained-release or long-acting. Sustained-release medications are used initially in pain management to control as much of the overall pain as possible. Pain episodes that occur despite good control of a sustained-release medication are called breakthrough pain. Medications that tend to give relief for 1 to 4 hours are called short-acting.

The least expensive opioid medication option is methadone. Many people are familiar with the name methadone because the drug is also used to help addicts to detoxify and stop using drugs illegally. But methadone is also used to treat pain, and its use in treating pain should not be confused with its use in addiction drug treatment. Methadone is also commonly prescribed in neuropathic pain states because of its additional ability to affect the NMDA receptor, or N-methyl-D-aspartic acid, the receptor that is believed to be involved in nerve pain states. Methadone is one of the trickiest opioids to prescribe. Because it affects pain for considerably less time than it is in the body, determining appropriate dosing is a challenge for health care providers.

One of the most effective opioids, oxycodone (OxyContin), has, unfortunately, become a popular drug among illegal drug users, and this creates problems. The more readily accessible an agent is, the more likely it is to be abused. Although addiction can occur with any narcotic, OxyContin is particularly appealing because it can be crushed or dissolved and then taken in multiple unintended ways—orally, nasally, or by intravenous injection. The formulation of this drug will be changed in the future to reduce its potential for abuse.

Tapentadol (Nucynta) is a new drug with opioid and nonopioid activity in a single compound. It is a centrally acting analgesic with a unique dual mode of action. Its potency is considered to be between morphine and tramadol.

When oral medications can't be used, fentanyl products administered trandermally—via a patch on the skin—are preferred. Duragesic is a sustained formulation of fentanyl that is slowly absorbed through the skin. Although some people metabolize drugs faster than others and may need to change their patch in two days, most patients find the patch can continually administer medication for three days. Duragesic comes in a branded and two generic forms; the rate fentanyl enters the body can differ between the products.

Actiq and Fentora provide another means to rapidly administer fentanyl to the body. The fast deliveries of these medications are a result of absorption through the buccal or inner cheek tissue of the mouth, and they can take effect in a matter of minutes. Actiq is fast; Fentora is faster. Other short-acting medications like Darvocet, Vicodin, or Percocet may take 45 minutes to start giving pain relief, whereas Actiq and Fentora may start to give analgesia within 15 minutes. At this time, Fentora is the most rapid means to administer fentanyl to the body without an invasive device, such as an IV, in an outpatient setting.

Morphine products like Avinza and Kadian are useful because they often need to be taken only once a day. Hydromorphone, or Dilaudid, often won't last as long as other class II opioids, but it generally has fewer side effects; an extended release formulation of this medication should be available in the near future. Oxymorphone, or Opana, is a potent narcotic favored for its ability to keep relatively constant the level of the medication entering and staying in the body.

There is a widespread preference in the pain management community for sustained-release medications. Typically these last 8 to 12 hours, or up to 72 hours with the patch, thereby reducing dosing frequency. This approach doesn't account for breakthrough pain, which can occur unexpectedly. Additionally, the need for medication can vary throughout the day. Many patients use a sustained-release medication combined with a rapid-action medicine for incidents that require additional control. I typically prescribe medications by considering what I would take if I had the pain problem myself. Some doctors call this the "your mama rule"—what would you give your mother if she had a pain problem. In general, I prefer a dose that would be sufficient to allow the completion of my various tasks that day without having to re-dose. If I needed a breakthrough medication, I would opt for the medication that would give me the fastest relief.

That said, there is no one perfect dose for everyone. A practitioner needs to individualize therapy for each patient. Some may do well with a sustained-release medication only. Others may need only a short-acting opioid for limited periods of time during the day. Many will need both.

Common Side Effects of Opioids

There are several potential side effects to opioids including constipation, nausea, vomiting, sedation, and itching. Some patients may experience decreased testosterone, which can lead to sexual dysfunction; there may be less drive for sexual activity among both male and female patients.

You may as well expect constipation with your first dose of a narcotic, because it is the most common side effect of opioids. Unfortunately, this annoyance may be a further aggravation of what patients are already experiencing with decreased motility from aging or an underlying associated disease such as diabetes. It's hard to assess what a "normal" bowel movement is, because it can vary greatly from person to person. For some, several bowel movements per day is normal and for others, one every three days is normal. If you are taking opioids and you have not had a bowel movement for more than four days, you should call your physician.

Patients will not usually become tolerant to opioid-induced constipation—that is, the constipation does not generally improve. While using opioids, you should be vigilant about drinking plenty of water and eating foods high in fiber. If this dietary regime is ineffective, it's time for a laxative.

Laxatives come in various forms, and one has not been proven better than another. I recommend trying the OTC—over-the-counter, no prescription needed—laxatives first, starting with Senokot S. Discuss all available OTC options with a pharmacist before pursuing prescription laxative therapy. If OTC therapy fails, ask your physician to provide a prescription for the drug Miralax. If Miralax doesn't give you relief, move on to orlistat (Alli), a diet pill that inhibits the absorption of one-third of the fat consumed; this medication is only effective if you consume high fatty meals, as most Americans do. Your physician might want to try one of the newer prescription treatments for constipation. Amitiza, a pill, alters the flow of chloride ions in the bowel wall so that fluid secretion in the intestines is increased, which in turn increases muscle movement in the intestine and helps make it easier to pass stools. Relistor (methyl-naltrexone) is an injectable that counteracts the narcotic effect on the bowel lumen but does not affect the potency of the narcotic in the central nervous system; in studies, bowel movements occurred 70 percent of the time.

If oral laxatives are ineffective, I recommend suppositories (rectally administered medicines) and only if suppositories are ineffective, I recommend enemas. If none of these remedies takes care of the problem, I recommend a bottle of magnesium citrate. And if nothing is effective, you must go to an emergency room for manual disimpaction, a process where a health care provider inserts a gloved finger into the rectum in order to dislodge stool. Most drug literature recommends limiting the use of laxatives; this recommendation does not apply to individuals using narcotics chronically. These individuals need to use laxatives regularly in order to prevent bowel problems.

Nausea is another possible side effect of taking opioids. When I was in medical school, the student lounge at the University of Maryland with its stale food smells was jokingly referred to as the area postrema, the area in the brain that causes nausea when stimulated. Opioids can stimulate the area postrema to cause nausea. That being said, there are several other reasons why one may become nauseated on opioids, including constipation and other medical illnesses.

Practitioners look at the timeline of nausea to help determine the reason for constipation. Nausea with a bowel movement suggests constipation; nausea soon after taking an opioid suggests it is medication induced. Some people find opioid-induced nausea worse than having pain itself. If nausea can be tolerated, this side effect may wane over a two-week period. During this brief period, or for other occasional bouts of nausea and vomiting, I recommend an antiemetic, such as hydroxyzine HCl, ondansetron, or prochlorperazine. Occasionally a person may need to take an antiemetic chronically, which may enhance the sedative properties of opioids.

If a particular opioid can't be tolerated, I recommend switching to another one, since nausea with one does not necessarily mean a patient will be nauseated with another.

Sleepiness is rarely seen in an opioid-tolerant patient, but tends to be more of an issue in the opioid naïve (that is, in a person who is newly taking opioids). Pain can counteract any soporific effects, however. If sedation is occurring, most people will become tolerant of it within two weeks. During this time, the patient may need to take a stimulant such as Provigil or Ritalin. Some few people will become chronically sedated on an opioid, in which case the patient and physician need to decide whether the benefits obtained from the narcotic outweigh the problem of sedation. Chronic sedation can also be treated with a stimulant or by altering the doses of other somnolent medications, lowering the dose of the opioid, and/or utilizing other interventions to decrease pain that will not be so sleep inducing.

You should not drive or operate machinery if your cognitive functions are impaired by opiate use. The good news is that several studies have shown that patients can use opioids chronically and still maintain normal cognitive function. However, these people were using a stable dose of medication and not mixing it with other systemic medications. If for work reasons or other reasons you need to prove that you can function on opioids, you should have the medication measured in your body with a serum and/or a urine test immediately preceding your driving test or functional capacity evaluation. These values can be referenced in the future as well.

Itching is another common side effect of opioids that usually becomes tolerable with time. This symptom commonly does not need to be treated. Itching that accompanies opioid use does not necessarily mean you are allergic to the medication; it usually is a manifestation of the effect of the narcotic on receptors in the body. If itching is persistent or bothersome, another opioid medication should be considered. The itching itself can be safely treated with Benadryl, hydroxyzine, or ondansetron.

Sexual dysfunction can occur with chronic use of narcotics. It is typically manifested by a lack of sexual drive. Some report a decreased zest for life. Testing for testosterone, the hormone typically affected by chronic narcotic use, can reveal if there is any insufficiency. For men, problems in sexual drive or functioning can be addressed with prescription medications available on the market such as testosterone injections, gels such as Androgel and Testim, and patches like Androderm. For women, a fraction of the dose used for men may be helpful.

Uncommon Side Effects of Opioids

Respiratory depression can occur if opioids are given too aggressively, so the dosing must be handled with great care. A physician needs to be especially cautious with opioids if the patient has respiratory disease such as pneumonia or sleep apnea. The respiratory limiting effect from the disease may be enhanced by the additional narcotic. If respiratory depression occurs, contact 911 for immediate medical care; *an overdose of a narcotic can lead to death.*

Also possible with opioid use is cognitive dysfunction, which usually decreases within the first two weeks of initiating opioid therapy. During those two weeks, however, the patient is impaired and should not drive. The condition can be further aggravated by other sedating medications such as alcohol or marijuana. At its most extreme, cognitive dysfunction may manifest itself as delirium, a problem sometimes seen in the very frail and terminally ill.

At high doses, all opioids can cause the spontaneous contraction of muscles, or myoclonus. Family members may notice that muscles are jerking at times. Decreasing the opioid dose or adding a muscle relaxant are reasonable therapeutic options.

Conditions Connected to Opioids

The use of opioids to manage chronic pain has not been universally accepted, and much ignorance and fear surround the subject. Understanding the terms below can help in the discussion.

Addiction refers to the continued use of a medication despite harm. Generally addiction occurs over time and is the byproduct of the interplay of genetics, environment, and drug exposure. A genetic predisposition to addiction would be suggested by a family history of substance abuse. A stressful environment at work, home, or in interpersonal relationships can also make someone more susceptible to developing the disease of addiction. An environmental predisposition refers to the people with whom one associates; if others condone substance abuse, you may be more likely to accept this behavior in yourself. A drug exposure predisposition refers to the access to narcotics whether through accepted channels (prescription of a medication by a doctor) or through ready access to illicit medications off the street. The universal medically reasonable use of opioids rarely leads to addiction. Using opioids does not necessarily mean someone is an addict. Most chronic pain patients who use opioids for pain management are not addicts.

Pseudoaddiction refers to behavior that mimics addiction but that resolves when adequate treatment of pain occurs.

Physical dependence refers to the necessary use of a medication for daily functioning. The hallmark of physical dependence is the development of withdrawal symptoms when a drug is abruptly stopped. Withdrawal symptoms occur with many different drugs including antihypertensive and antidepressant medications. The withdrawal of opioids can cause flulike symptoms when physical dependence has occurred. Physical dependency does not mean addiction; withdrawal is a physiologic response to long-term exposure to many types of drugs.

Tolerance refers to when a medicine loses its effectiveness over time. A different, often stronger, agent is needed in order to obtain the desired effect. This effect is not unique to opioids but also occurs with insulin and many heart medications. If a patient becomes "tolerant" of a particular medicine, it does not mean he is addicted to it.

What a Physician Considers When Prescribing Opioids

Physicians prescribing opioids for a chronic condition (and therefore for an indefinite period of time) must consider several issues. Some patients will have an increased risk of developing problems while on these medications, most notably people with a prior history of abuse of illicit or licit substances (such as alcohol); those with a history of physical or sexual abuse; and individuals with active psychiatric diseases.

If a person has an increased chance of having problems with opioids, it's a good idea for the physician to prescribe psychological guidance as a complementary therapy. Doctors may want to screen patients prior to opioid use by means of a urine and serum drug test, both to verify the patient's history and to offer guidance for his or her subsequent care. An opioid agreement may also be presented that spells out expectations and helps ensure that these expectations are clearly understood by all parties involved in the treatment.

An opioid agreement usually outlines some of the responsibilities that the patient agrees to assume if controlled substances are prescribed. For example, the patient will usually be asked not to obtain controlled substances from any other physician, not to share drugs with others, and to take the medication only as prescribed. There are often other responsibilities as well that the patient agrees to accept in order to embark on long-term opioid therapy; these responsibilities are designed to make the use of these powerful drugs as safe as possible. For example, it is important to keep these medicines out of the reach of children or other adults, which can be accomplished by using a locked cabinet or a safe.

When opioids are prescribed, it is with the physician's expectation of functional improvement. Improvement will mean different things to each patient. For a person in bed 20 hours a day because of pain, improved function may mean performing activities around the house for half the day. For those prevented from working because of their pain, it may mean a return to work. Even with these functional goals in mind, the health care practitioner needs to continually assess the appropriate use of these medications in relation to the patient's needs.

The Pros and Cons of Opioid Treatment

Though not in every study, on the whole, opioids have been scientifically shown to decrease suffering in many chronic pain conditions. Corresponding to this relief is improved functionality, which happens more often than not. Most people are elated to find something that helps with their discomfort and many respond accordingly by becoming more active and more engaged in life.

Opioids do not solve all chronic pain problems; some patients do not achieve pain relief from opioids. And opioids may reduce pain but not improve function. As a practitioner, my goal is to see both reduced pain and improved function. Patients must understand that maximum pain relief may not produce maximum function. If you are taking so much medication that you are in a stupor, then your functional level is poor. You may have less pain but still not be able to participate in family life, do chores, or be actively engaged in life. As a pain physician, I would tell you that we need to reduce the dose of the medication to allow you to become more functional and that we will address the increased pain through other therapeutic options.

All opioids have the potential to cause addiction. That being said, very few people actually become addicted. As noted above, addiction depends upon many variables, and if a patient is not at risk owing to genetic, social, and psychiatric factors, his or her chances of becoming addicted to a narcotic are low. The American Society of Addiction Medicine estimates that 10 percent of the general population is at risk of developing the disease of opioid addiction when exposed to opioids chronically. People with genetic, social, or psychiatric factors predisposing them to addiction may have a 50 percent risk of becoming addicted if they use opioids chronically. Therefore, people at greater risk may not be good candidates for opioids.

Topicals | Pain medication applied to the skin

The main pain reliever in the class of topical medications is a Lidocaine patch 5 percent, or Lidoderm. This 10 × 14 cm patch releases a local anesthetic continuously. The patient applies it in the morning and removes it in the evening. Its only FDA indication is for postherpetic neuralgia (herpes-related nerve pain). In practice, people try this medication for many different pains. It is very well tolerated and its most common side effect is local skin irritation. An early study showed some promise for its use in patients with low back pain. If a back pain area can be covered with your two hands, then this may be an agent to try.

Flector Patch, available only by prescription, releases a nonsteroidal anti-inflammatory medication through the skin. The patch may be used to treat acute and local inflammatory conditions such as minor sprains, strains, and bruises, but it is not indicated for treatment of chronic low back pain.

There are many formulations of topical compounds that can be produced, such as: clonidine, capsaicin, ketamine, amitriptyline, gabapentin, and nonsteroidals. However, these medications have not been studied or examined in enough patients to be widely accepted as topicals and used in the pain management arena.

Patches are prescribed by a doctor. Creams are available over the counter in pharmacies or in compounding pharmacies (whose pharmacists will compound custom medications for the needs of the specific patient).

Antidepressants | Because depression and pain are linked

Depression can magnify the perception of pain. The majority of people with chronic pain exhibit some symptoms of depression. There are similar pathways for depression and pain in the central nervous system. Treating depression can help reduce the perception of pain; treating pain can help reduce depression. Antidepressants are used not only to help with depression but also because they have been shown to reduce pain when no depression is present (one antidepressant with this effect is Cymbalta). Or, because they induce sleepiness, some antidepressants may help those with chronic pain who also suffer from insomnia.

There are many classes of antidepressants. They are classified according to their chemical structures or the neurotransmitters they inhibit. One class you may have heard of, monoamine oxidase inhibitors (MAOIs), are rarely prescribed for pain management and are not discussed here.

Tricyclic antidepressants (TCAs) (classified by chemical structure)
amitriptyline (elavil)
desipramine (Norpramin)
doxepin (Sinequan)
imipramine (Tofranil)
nortriptyline (Aventyl, Pamelor)
protriptyline (Vivactil)

Selective serotonin reuptake inhibitors (SSRIs) (the neurotransmitter
   serotonin is inhibited)
citalopram (Celexa)
fluoxetine (Prozac, Sarafem)
fluvoxamine (Luvox)
paroxetine (Paxil)
sertraline (Zoloft)

Serotonin-norepinephrine reuptake inhibitors (SNRIs) (the neurotransmitters serotonin and norepinephrine are inhibited)
bupropion (Wellbutrin)
duloxetine (Cymbalta)
maprotiline (Ludiomil)
mirtazapine (Remeron)
nefazodone (Serzone)
trazodone (Desyrel)
venlafaxine (Effexor)

TCAs have been shown to help many people with chronic pain. Treatment is inexpensive, typically a few dollars for a day of medication. Their chief downside is their side effects. Each TCA agent appears comparable in efficacy, but varies in its potential adverse reactions, which can include sleepiness, weight gain, blurry vision, dry mouth, constipation, and urinary hesitancy. There is a narrow therapeutic window for use of these medicines, which means that a specific serum concentration needs to be obtained to get the desired effect—too low a concentration produces no effect and too high a concentration results in overmedication. An excess of these medications (overdose) has led to fatal arrythmias and death. Though unintended consequences can occur with the first dose of medication, a person often develops tolerance for the side effects over the first two weeks. Tolerating side effects can mean either that the patient learns to live with the side effects or that the patient no longer experiences them.

A beneficial reduction in pain usually is observed before the improvement in depression, but neither may be noted for as long as four to six weeks. No clear guidelines on the doses needed to obtain pain relief have been published, but in my own experience there is a significant variability in analgesic doses between patients. TCAs are not recommended for elderly people because of the side effect profile and because of the frequency of other diseases such as cardiovascular disease that affect people over the age of 65.

Randomized, double-blind, placebo-controlled studies in patients with chronic low back pain without depression showed significant pain reduction in patients using nortriptyline (a TCA) or maprotiline (an SNRI), but not paroxetine (an SSRI). The mixed agents (SNRIs) tend to have fewer side effects than the tricyclic antidepressants (TCAs). None of the SSRIs has conclusively proven to be helpful in reducing chronic low back pain.

Using SSRIs for pain treatment has shown mixed scientific results. Recently, a study at the University of California at San Francisco showed high-dose Prozac (60 mg/day) reduced pain in patients with postherpetic neuralgia (herpes-related nerve pain).[1] One can extrapolate from this well-done study that Prozac may also help people with neuropathic low back pain. One out of three people who uses these agents develops sexual dysfunction in the form of decreased libido, impotence, ejaculatory disturbances, or anorgasmia (inability to reach orgasm). Sexual dysfunction problems related to the medications resolve when the person stops taking the medication.

Prozac and Zoloft tend to be more activating and therefore should be taken in the morning. Lexapro is neutral. Paxil tends to sedate and therefore should be dosed in the evening prior to bed.

Many of my patients have expressed concern that taking an antidepressant somehow implies that their pain is all in their head. Antidepressants have enhanced the quality of life for many people with chronic low back pain, and there's no reason for patients to deprive themselves of this relief if they fall into this group. Follow your physician's advice.

Sixty percent of individuals who take an antidepressant for depression will experience improvement, regardless of the medication used. There are some specific guidelines I follow, however, in choosing the right antidepressant for a patient. I usually do not recommend TCAs for anyone with cardiac or seizure history. TCAs lower the arrhythmia and seizure threshold, making these events more likely to occur. TCAs can cause anticholinergic effects, such as sedation, blurred vision, urinary retention, or constipation. I avoid TCAs in the frail and those over 65 years of age because those patients tend not to tolerate this class of medication very well. Last, but not least, there is a significant weight gain issue with TCAs; many people will have an increased interest in sugars. When TCAs are used, I prefer to use the lowest doses, starting at 10 mg and adjusting weekly while the patient develops a tolerance to the side effects. I find this approach helps more patients adhere to the medicine regimen.

A person can overdose with TCAs; this is a lot less likely to occur with the SSRIs and SNRIs. Abruptly stopping the TCAs can lead to a withdrawal syndrome. SNRIs are the newest antidepressants and have the lowest side-effect profile. Wellbutrin, however, should not be used by people with seizures or eating disorders or by people taking MAOIs (monoamine oxidase inhibitors), another class of inhibitors.

One antidepressant, Cymbalta, has been clinically proven to help with the chronic pain state of painful diabetic peripheral neuropathy as well as depression and anxiety, and it is generally well tolerated. In addition, people who take this medication generally do not gain weight and it does not appear to have much of an effect on an individual's sexual function.

The TCA elavil has the best ratio for "numbers-needed-to-treat" before an observed response of all the antidepressants. "Numbers-needed-to-treat" refers to the proportion of how many patients getting a medication will respond to it; for elavil it is approximately one out of three. Nevertheless, I still exercise great caution with TCAs.

The SNRI trazodone is the most sedating of all the antidepressants and is the treatment most often prescribed for insomnia in chronic pain patients. A prolonged painful erection, a condition known as priapism, is a rare but notable side effect with this drug.

Just because you don't respond to one antidepressant does not mean you should give up on all of them. Typically two or more agents need to be tried before finding one that works for you. Do not take a monoamine oxidase inhibitor (MAOI) such as phenelzine with another antidepressant. Antidepressants were formulated to treat depression, so we do not have a complete grasp of their full benefits on chronic low back pain.

Antiepileptics | Drugs that suppress epilepsy

Many antiepileptic medications have been shown in studies to help relieve neuropathic pain states—pain that is the byproduct of either damage or dysfunction in the nervous system. These drugs modulate nerve function while allowing the nerves to continue to send signals; pain can be blocked in a nerve while the same nerve still functions in sending information. It must be kept in mind that success with one of these agents does not predict success with another. Options include:

carbamazepine (Carbatrol, Tegretol)
clonazepam (Klonopin)
divalproex sodium (Depakote)
gabapentin (Neurontin)
lamotrigine (Lamictal)
levetiracetam (Keppra)
phenytoin (Dilantin)
pregabalin (Lyrica)
oxcarbazepine (Trileptal)
tiagabine (Gabitril)
topiramate (Topamax)
valproic acid (Depakene)
zonisamide (Zonegran)

These medications are generally well tolerated with minimal side effects, such as dizziness, somnolence (sleepiness), ataxia (lack of coordination), and peripheral edema (swelling of the arms or legs). Neurontin and Lyrica work by affecting calcium channel functioning on nerves (more on this in a moment). These drugs stabilize nerve membranes and help reduce unwanted activation or firing of irritable nerves; the result is seen as a reduction in seizures in the brain and a decrease in pain from injured nerves. Until recently, Neurontin was my first choice for treating neuropathic pain because it had minimal effect on other drugs. A physician can rapidly increase the dose of the medication until a response is obtained, an intolerable side effect is produced, or the maximum amount that can be absorbed is reached (3600 mg/day). Recently I have changed my primary antiepileptic of choice to treat neuropathic pain to Lyrica. Lyrica appears to have a similar side-effect profile to Neurontin, but in some studies it has been shown to be more effective; for many people, the initial starting dose (150 mg) will be effective.

Other Nerve Channel Modulators | Controlling other pain paths

Sodium and calcium channels exist on nerves in both the central and peripheral nervous systems. These channels are active when nerves are working normally. In chronic pain states it is thought that many of these channels increase in number and change in function and, in fact, may become too active in neuropathic pain states. The following medicines modulate these channels and therefore have a potential effect on neuropathic pain:

> lidocaine (Lidoderm)
> mexiletine (Mexitil)
> ziconotide (Prialt)

These agents are not often used in pain management, though some experimental results suggest they may be promising. Part of the reason for restraint in using these medications is the lack of experience and a fear of potential problems. We know, however, that lamotrigine not only helps with pain but has a mood-stabilizing effect. Ziconotide appears promising but not widely used because the medication is expensive and a surgical procedure must be done to implant an intrathecal pump to deliver it.

Muscle Relaxants | To relax painful muscle spasms

Many chronic low back pain states are accompanied by muscle spasms. Most muscle relaxants do more to relax the brain than the muscles. Most of the drugs in this class have a primary sedative quality; in general, these drugs do not really have a direct effect on muscles. Valium is used in clinical practice more for anxiety, yet it can be a great muscle relaxant during the acute phases of muscle injury. Quinine is a membrane stabilizer also used to treat malaria. Baclofen is a good drug that can be used orally but works better spinally; however, seizures are a risk with abrupt withdrawal. Flexeril has properties in common with the TCAs. Botox and Prialt are two examples of the interesting phenomenon of using select toxins to make useful drugs. Muscles can be relaxed, and pain can often be reduced, by using the following agents, known as muscle relaxants:

baclofen (Lioresal)
carisoprodol (Soma)
chlorzoxazone (Parafon Forte)
cyclobenzaprine (Flexeril, Amrix)
dantrolene (Dantrium)
diazepam (Valium)
metaxalone (Skelaxin)
methocarbamol (Robaxin)
orphenadrine (Norflex)
quinine (Qualaquin)
tizanidine (Zanaflex)

Botox is an injectable agent that can also be considered a muscle relaxant. One injection can affect a muscle for three months.

There is no evidence to prove one branded medicine relaxes muscles better than another. The most commonly prescribed muscle relaxant is cyclobenzaprine. Amrix is the only available once-a-day formulation of cyclobenzaprine; in this form it offers a known muscle relaxant with the convenience of daily dosing. Zanaflex offers flexible dosing, but it should not be taken by anyone with liver dysfunction. The dose ranges from one to nine pills in a day.

All muscle relaxants cause some level of sedation. This can be helpful at night when people want to sleep but problematic during the day when they need to function. Quinine is the treatment of choice for nighttime leg cramps.

Other Types of Drugs | Not primarily intended for pain relief

Cannabinoids (Marijuana). Some preliminary studies have shown that medicinal marijuana has therapeutic promise. In addition to analgesia, it has properties as an antiemetic and appetite stimulant. However, studies have not been extensive enough to win over the scientific community. In addition, it is a controlled substance, and its regulatory control dissuades most clinicians from considering it.

Benzodiazepines are the treatment of choice for most anxiety states; psychiatrists typically are the largest prescribers of this class of medication. Anxiety can magnify pain, yet it is common in people with chronic pain and it becomes an issue when it impairs function.

In the pain clinic, the benzodiazepine agents are usually reserved for acute pain situations. (One exception is clonazepam, or Klonopin, which is both a benzodiazepine and an antiepileptic drug.) When a person has acute pain, diazepam (Valium, which is both a benzodiazepine and a muscle relaxant) can be helpful in reducing muscle spasms and relieving anxiety. Clonazepam may help with muscle spasms and has been shown to be useful in treating neuropathic pain. Part of the problem with continued use of these medicines is a risk of memory impairment and learning problems. Other problems include sedation, confusion, agitation, respiratory depression, and, potentially, death from overdose. Abruptly stopping the medicines in this class could lead to seizures and/or death. *If you want to stop using these medications, slowly wean yourself from them over a several-week period, with the advice of your physician.*

Hydroxyzine (Vistaril), an antihistamine, has been shown to have some intrinsic analgesic activity. Nevertheless, it is usually used with other medications to reduce nausea.

Amphetamines are commonly used to counteract medication-induced sedation and treat attention deficit disorders. Although amphetamines have never been shown to have any intrinsic analgesic activity, some studies suggest they can enhance the effects of opioid analgesia.

This chapter has reviewed the many medications used to treat low back pain. In addition to or in place of prescription medicines, your doctor may also recommend pharmaceuticals that are designed to work in pinpointed areas of the body and that are delivered at the doctor's office or in the clinic. These treatments are covered in the next chapter.

Chapter 8
Injections and Other Treatments

By targeting the point of pain, a well-placed injection can bring welcome relief.

DETERMINING THE CAUSE OF back pain can be difficult. In some circumstances, an injection of local anesthetic into the spine helps to *locate* the source of the pain. If the ensuing numbness eliminates the pain, then the physician may infer that he or she is in the right area. In this case, the injection has been used as a *diagnostic* tool. Injections are used to *treat* back pain, too, in which case a steroid or Botox is injected into the spine as a *therapeutic* tool. A physician should not consider treating a patient with an injection into the spine unless there is evidence to support the belief that the area intended for injection is likely the source of the problem. Prior evaluations should have verified that the site is the most likely origin of the pain and that the description of pain reported by the patient matches the kind of discomfort typically felt at that site.

Injection therapy should be considered only after other reasonable interventions—such as activity modification and physical therapy—have been tried. Although injections can be diagnostic and therapeutic, the results of injections can be difficult to interpret accurately. Even though it is possible for a single treatment to provide relief, most people will still need a multidisciplinary approach to bring about lasting change in their back pain.

Injections may also be considered if the site of pain is still not clearly identified after physical and radiographic studies. If pain improves after injection, it's possible that the area injected is the source of the pain (but not always; see below). This is why injection is sometimes simultaneously diagnostic and therapeutic.

Radiographs, such as x-rays, CT scans, MRIs, bone scans, SPECT scans, and PET scans, show anatomy but do not reveal whether a particular point is in distress. Only the patient can confirm whether pain exists in that area. Electromyograms and nerve conduction tests, known as EMG/NCS, are helpful in revealing abnormalities in motor and sensory neurons, but they may not be the source of the problem. In other words, a patient could have a normal EMG/NCS and have pain nevertheless.

Interpreting Injections | Did it get to the source of the pain?

Potential sites for injections include nerve roots, facet joints, sacroiliac joints, and discs. While valuable diagnostic information can be obtained via injections, confounding factors can muddy the results. Let's say anesthetizing "area X" of the spine with injection leads to relief, suggesting it is the source of pain. This is a logical assumption, but it may not be completely true. Was "area X" truly anesthetized, or was neighboring "structure Y" affected too? If so, is "Y" the true culprit? The correct answer is crucial because surgeons might be relying on it for information about where to operate. If they treat the incorrect area, the patient winds up being no better after surgery. Injections used to determine the source of pain have been estimated to be correct only 50 percent of the time—and approximately 75 percent of chronic low back pain has an undiagnosed source.

There is also the possibility that the injection was not performed perfectly. The doctor may have intended to inject "X," but since it is so close to "Y," that may be where the insertion in fact took place. Subsequent treatment of "X" with no response could indicate not that the treatment is ineffective, but that the wrong area is being addressed. To improve accuracy, fluoroscopy or a CT scan should be used. Another pitfall with injections is that more than one area may be contributing to the pain. Maybe "X" *and* "Y" are the culprits. A partial response at "area X" may lead to dismissing it as a source of pain—likewise for "Y"—yet it could really mean that more than one infusion is needed to clarify the condition completely. A lack of response could also indicate that the tip of the needle went into a vascular structure, such as a vein or artery, instead of its intended target, the spine. In that case, the injected medicine would immediately be transported away from the area identified for treatment. This pitfall can be avoided by using dye in the injection, which maps the exact route of the medicine.

The placebo effect is another potential problem with injections. Derived from Greek, placebo means "I will please," and when used in reference to medication, it implies that the patient's desire to be better is making him or her report wellness that may not, in fact, exist. Patients typically want to please their practitioner; they also want to feel better. Their hope for cure, combined with a faith that their doctor can solve their problem if only they believe hard enough, is a recipe for the placebo effect. This cycle can muddy interpretation of the results.

To clarify the source of pain via injection, multiple areas should be injected and the results viewed together. An injection can be repeated to see if it elicits a similar response the second time, a process that may reveal a placebo responder. Another approach is to perform two insertions, one with an inactive agent. The patient who is a "placebo responder" is likely to react to both injections, whereas the normal responder would perceive an effect only with the active agent.

Somewhat related to placebo pain is the "referred pain" response (see below). In referred pain, the problem is in one location, the back for instance, but is perceived in another site, like the leg. Doctors are familiar with the concept of referred pain but can be misled if they rely on the response to only one injection.

Additionally, since it takes approximately two days for the effect of steroid injections to be manifested, any other treatments the patient is using—physical therapy, painkillers, and so on—can cause the results to be unclear. Did the person improve because of the injected steroid or because of the physical therapy? Maybe—even likely—both contributed. Furthermore, steroids are absorbed systemically, so an injection at "area X," even dye-confirmed, could be absorbed by "area Y" and affect "Y" just as readily as "X." There are also dosing issues with steroids.

Trigger Point Injections | Easy, popular, and usually safe

The back contains not only the spine but many supporting structures: ligaments, tendons, muscle, and fascia, which is the "glue" that keeps it altogether. These extra spinal structures can be the source of pain. Through a physical exam, the doctor can typically locate the sensitive area or areas. This site, the trigger point, when touched, may cause pain to radiate into another area, which is called *referred pain*. Pathologically, the tissue may appear normal. In this example, the patient is considered to have myofascial pain or a spinal enthesopathy. We don't know how common spinal enthesopathy is, but the literature suggests that more women than men have this problem.

Trigger points are discrete taut bands in muscle. They may be felt with or without movement, or they may be activated only when touched. They may be the only source of the problem or a small piece of a more complicated puzzle. Muscle pain can also indicate a systemic disease: thyroid problems, electrolyte abnormalities, neurologic disease, or autoimmune disease. Failure to differentiate a systemic disease from an enthesopathy or spinal disease can lead to a prolonged and unsuccessful therapy.

Once the systemic diseases have been ruled out, it's time to look at enthesopathy. This type of problem is usually localized in one area of the back rather than felt in the whole body. Typically there is a taut muscle. Occasionally the physician can find a hyperexcitable area in the muscle. If this area becomes desensitized after the injection of local anesthetic, the physician has identified a trigger point—but this is a hard thing to do in a spasming muscle.

Treatment of a trigger point starts with some kind of functional enhancement, typically physical therapy. If the area is too painful for manipulation, medications or injections should be used to allow the patient to exercise the area. Injection involves first identifying the trigger point, then passing a needle through the skin into the point; this is typically done multiple times. It is thought that the needle entering the trigger point stimulates a local inflammatory reaction, which leads to a positive change.

I inject local anesthetic because patients tell me they like the way the muscle feels afterward. During the procedure, some stretching manipulation of the area can be done, and a skin coolant can be applied to enhance muscle relief. After the treatment, the patient should be able to use the muscle. If the trigger point becomes problematic again, reinjection can be done. What physicians like to see happen is increased periods of relief with each intervention; for example, the first shot may result in only one day of relief, while the second may give three days, and so forth. If the periods of relief don't increase, I would consider other methods. There is no exact number of injections one can perform, although some insurance plans limit the number that can be performed over a one-year period, and most physicians recommend limiting the number of injections to three within a six-month period. The physician's judgment is the ultimate guide.

If the above injection methods don't yield satisfactory results, it's time to move on to Botox injections, whose full effects are typically noticed within two weeks. Botox is a trademark name for a chemical preparation of botulinum toxin, a chemical that can paralyze muscle for approximately three months. There is also a belief that it alters pain-signaling chemicals in the spinal cord. With the expected relief, the patient can then pursue more aggressive physical therapy. The hope is that by the time the Botox has worn off, the patient has improved function, and the change resulting from PT will mean that no further treatment is needed. That said, many people still need repeat injections. The attraction of Botox is the prolonged relief with a single dose. The biggest shortcoming is cost: two trigger point treatments can run $1,000, and insurance companies are reluctant to cover Botox treatments outside its FDA-approved uses: strabismus, blepharospasm, hemifacial spasm, and cervical dystonia.

Trigger point injections are among the easiest to perform and the most common used by physicians for pain. It is rare to have a complication from this intervention, but problems have occurred: hematoma (bruise), infection, allergic reaction, nerve injury, and adjacent organ trauma. It is imperative to add exercise to this approach for lasting effect.

If trigger point injections are ineffective, the physician could turn to muscle stimulation, which involves using therapeutic pads on the skin where symptoms are occurring. Electricity moves from one pad to another. Treatments typically last 20 minutes and may be done up to four times a day. If a patient gets successful results, he or she can purchase the device. Reduction of symptoms should be accompanied by increased function. Typically insurance companies will purchase the device for patients who have completed a trial with it and have noted significant benefit. Muscle stimulation differs from TENS, discussed in chapter 5, in the depth of the electrical waves traveling into the body.

Spinal Injections | Taking therapy to the next level

If the muscular and soft tissue explanation for low back pain has been resolved and the problem persists, it's time to consider whether the problem is coming from one of the following three structures: facet joints, sacroiliac joints, or discs. The history and physical exam will direct the doctor to the suspected pain source, but when the source of pain can't be determined, the doctor will start with the easiest injection to perform—facets—and progress to the most difficult—discs—until the source is identified. Forty percent of chronic low back pain probably derives from these structures, with the incidence more common in older patients.

Facet Injections

Facets are two of the three joints that exist between vertebrae; the other contains a disc. A facet, or zygapophyseal joint, is a synovial joint that can degenerate like any other body part. As the back ages, these structures become more stressed, and when degeneration such as arthritis is added, this area becomes an increasing source of pain. However, the presence of arthritis does not necessarily mean that this is the cause of the distress. The pain produced by these structures is typically located in the back and occasionally radiates into the buttocks, hips, and legs, above the knees. It may occur on only one side of the back. It can be established that a facet is causing the problem if the pain goes away after the joint is anesthetized. History and physical exam do not reliably identify whether the facet is the source of pain.

Facet disease must be considered when back trauma with resulting pain is experienced but radiographic findings remain normal. Another sign of facet disease is back pain that is responsive to chiropractic manipulation. Problems with these joints can occur if they are adjacent—a transitional facet—to a part of the back that had been fused at one time with the normal spine. The stress of the fused area gets transferred to the transitional facet area.

Facet injections must be performed with radiographic guidance from either fluoroscopy or CT scan. This procedure should not be performed on patients with an active systemic infection, a bleeding predisposition, or those who are pregnant. Patients on blood thinners should contact their primary physician to inquire about the appropriateness and timing for this medication, and people with diabetes should be aware that steroids can increase serum glucose for up to two weeks. Any patient with an artificial heart valve should contact his or her primary care physician to inquire whether antibiotic prophylaxis is warranted.

To receive a facet injection, the patient lies prone, face down, and a needle is advanced through the skin to the joint. Local anesthetic and/or a steroid are injected. Usually within 30 minutes the patient will respond to the injection. To qualify as facet disease, the patient should have repeated therapeutic results to this treatment. As noted, many insurance companies allow three injections of steroids to be performed into the same joint over a twelve-month period. If the patient does not obtain a satisfactory response to steroids, the physician may consider a procedure in which the nerve endings entering the facets are ablated with radiofrequency waves (RF). If there is no lasting effect, referral to a surgeon for a possible fusion of the joint should be considered.

RF involves the insertion of an "introducer" at the facet. An introducer is an insulated needle that has an exposed tip to allow radiofrequency waves to be emitted. A probe is inserted through the introducer and attached to a box that administers the treatment. A sensory stimulation pattern occurs, and the physician asks the patient where he or she feels stimulation; if it's in the area where the patient typically feels pain, then the practitioner will proceed with the testing. A motor stimulation test involves stimulating the area of treatment to see if a motor nerve reacts. RF destroys nerve tissue, and no one wants to lose motor nerves. Once this testing is completed, treatment starts. The effect from an RF may not be realized for as long as a month, although no one knows why.

If a facet has been correctly identified as a source of the problem and a proper RF procedure has been performed, we can expect a 50 percent reduction in low back pain to last approximately two years. The procedure causes the involved nerve endings to burn, and since these ultimately grow back, the treatment is not a permanent cure. It is also possible to experience a worsening of pain for a period of time—possibly weeks—after an RF. There is also the possibility of affecting nerve function in nerves not targeted to be altered. For the most part, however, RF is considered a very safe procedure.

Sacroiliac Injections

Approximately 15 percent of chronic low back pain emanates from the sacroiliac joint.. There are many ways to evaluate this joint, but none is reliable for verifying it as a source of pain. Radiographs such as a plain x-ray, bone scans, SPECT, CT, and MRI may show changes or abnormalities, but these also do not prove that the sacroiliac joint is the culprit. The gold standard for diagnosis is local anesthetic; if the back pain resolves once local anesthetic is injected, the problem lies in the sacroiliac joint.

A synovial joint attaches the spine to the pelvis and is considered very strong. It contains a variety of ligaments, muscle, and tissue and functions in conjunction with the base of the spine, as well as the corresponding hip. A series of nerves both in front and behind connect the joint to the spine and account for the variety of descriptions of referred pain from this joint, as well as the difficulty in identifying and treating sacroiliac pain.

Typically patients report pain in the buttock area that does not radiate into the leg. The first approach to this problem is always physical therapy, with the goal to restore muscle balance in the joint area. Some health professionals use orthotics (shoe inserts) to treat the joint, supporting the weak and ineffective muscles, but there have been insufficient studies to validate this approach. Others believe that manipulation of the joint can lead to relief, but this is another approach that has insufficient scientific corroboration. When conservative measures for treatment have failed, injections of the joint should be considered.

Injections of the sacroiliac require radiographic assistance such as fluoroscopy or CT scan to provide visualization for proper placement of the medication. The patient lies prone for the procedure as a small needle is advanced into the joint. The dye helps confirm the correct positioning of the needle, which will deliver local anesthetic and/or steroid. Typically, within 30 minutes a response is noted. As mentioned before, a single injection will not provide a definitive conclusion. Also as stated earlier, physical therapy should always be undertaken to enhance function.

If repeat injections and physical therapy are ineffective in providing the desired relief, RF may be considered. In this procedure, an introducer is placed at multiple sites along the joint, and nerve endings into the joint are treated to create lesions. This treatment is considered controversial. No significant outcome studies on RF of the sacroiliac have been produced, but in my practice it appears that 50 percent of people receiving the treatment (after obtaining short-term relief with local anesthetics and steroids) experience 50 percent pain relief for six months. Typically, repeat lesioning will be required in the future because nerve fibers grow back.

Only if physical therapy, steroid injections, and RF have failed would I consider other options like prolotherapy, neuromodulation, and surgery. Prolotherapy involves the injection of an agent (such as glucose) into the joint to promote inflammation with the belief that this inflammation will lead to pain reduction. Neuromodulation means the placement of a surgical lead over nerves in the spine in order to alter the signals going to the brain. To fuse the joint to keep it from moving requires surgery. All these options have their proponents but insufficient scientific evidence exists about their success.

Intervertebral Disc Injections

Only when facet and sacroiliac joint treatments have not helped should one consider the evaluation of discs. Forty percent of chronic low back pain derives from discs. Plain radiographs, CT scans, MRIs, and myelography make it possible to picture these structures but do not reveal whether they are painful. A discogram, during which dye is injected into the injured disc or discs to make the disc more visible in an x-ray, is the only way to clarify whether a disc is the source of the problem.

The disc is composed of two structures: the nucleus pulposus and the annulus fibrosis (see the appendix for a complete description and illustration). The former works as the shock absorber for the spine and has a high content of water; the latter, composed of tough tissue, keeps the vertebrae from moving too much. Studies have shown nerve endings in the annulus fibrosis.

Quite simply, as one ages, the spine degenerates. Degeneration is a fact of life and is associated with the loss of elasticity. In the disc, degeneration is manifested by the loss of hydration in the nucleus pulposus. The disc may appear to sag and show changes like herniations. The degenerative process results in discs that are less able to handle stress and more likely to sustain tears. Chemicals within the disc can escape through these fissures and irritate nerves in the back. To clarify which of the discs is the offending one, a discogram should be performed.

As with every spinal injection procedure, risks are present, including bleeding, allergic reaction, and, more importantly, infection and nerve injury. Infection occurs in approximately five out of a thousand procedures; it can be very difficult to treat and usually requires some time in the hospital to resolve. If there is a chance of infection, usually because of a less than robust immune system—as a consequence of either disease or medications—then antibiotics should be taken beforehand. The risk of nerve injury is due to the possibility that the needle is not appropriately placed into the disc. A patient needs to be alert during needle advancement to let the doctor know if any paresthesia occurs (paresthesia is the perception of an electrical shock, or a "pins and needles" feeling, flowing into the leg). Nerve injury is rare.

Fluoroscopy or CT is used to guide the placement of the needles, which are inserted into all joints to be studied. Pressure is applied to the plunger of a needle and if there are no contraindications, dye is injected. Contraindications are factors that make a drug or a procedure inadvisable. Contraindications to spinal injections include localized infection in the area identified for injection, systemic infections, irregularities in blood coagulation, and a medically unstable patient.

The questions posed to the patient during the procedure may include the following:

- What do you feel?
- Where do you feel it?
- How is this similar to the pain that brought you here?
- Is the quality of the pain similar to your typical experience?
- How would you rate the intensity of your discomfort?

To prevent skewed results, the patient should not be told what dosages are being injected, and each site should be injected twice to verify consistency. Usually a permanent radiographic image is obtained at the end of the procedure. For most physicians, a fluoroscopic image is sufficient but some may obtain a CT scan. If all the discs hurt, then there is no one site on which to focus therapy. In this case, the entire back must be treated. For patients with identifiably painful discs, specific therapy can be offered, both nonsurgical and surgical.

Over the past twenty years, the practice of removing disc material without surgically opening the body has evolved in procedures such as chemonucleolysis, percutaneous manual nucleotomy, thermal vaporization with a laser, and nucleotomy using Coblation technology, known as nucleoplasty. Each reduces pressure by removing some of the nucleus volume of the disc and involves few complications when performed by experienced hands. If this approach is unsuccessful, a surgical discectomy (removal of the entire disc) can be pursued.

Another way to change the disc is by altering the annulus fibrosis. Since nerve endings exist in this part of the disc, various types of energy, such as laser or electrical or radiofrequency, can be used to ablate the nerve endings, or the disc can be surgically removed or altered. Studies have produced mixed results in their support of percutaneous disc procedures. The lack of a large amount of data has kept these techniques from being covered by many insurance plans and accepted as a logical step in care. But these approaches are now actively being studied, since they pose a low risk compared to surgery.

Epidural Injections

Performed for more than fifty years, one of the most common injections for back pain is the epidural. The name refers to the space in the spine where the medicine is injected, a spot between the spinal cord and nerve rootlets and the bony part of the spinal column. Part of the nerve, the dorsal root ganglion (DRG), resides in this area. The intent of an epidural is to alter the pathology occurring at this site, primarily with steroids. The closer the physician can get the medicine to the target, the more likely it is that there will be a change in the patient's pain.

The problems at this site are not completely understood but are thought to include inflammation that leads to low back pain and associated radicular pain (pain in the back that radiates to other areas like the buttocks, thighs, hamstrings, or calves). Many inflammatory cytokines, that is, proteins that communicate between cells, have been identified as being active here, and there may be varying degrees of mechanical compression from disc material.

Steroids act by disrupting the inflammation, with subsequent healing at the site. The disc in the area may not change at all. Steroids also reduce nerve swelling, which is typically associated with inflammation, and blunt the activity of nerve fibers in the area. Local anesthetics injected during the procedure can help for a short period, one to six hours, in breaking the cycle of pain.

An epidural is primarily performed on patients having pain in their back that radiates into their legs, a condition referred to as sciatica. Fortunately, most sciatica will resolve without treatment within four weeks. Many people with only low back pain are also injected. In this circumstance, the injection is best at the onset of the pain, when there are concurrent dysfunction and behavioral changes. Otherwise, low back pain should initially be addressed with conservative interventions that primarily help in controlling the symptoms within a month of onset; if relief has not occurred, then an epidural should be considered.

Epidurals have been shown to offer all sorts of benefits: pain can be reduced; function can be restored; physical rehab can be started sooner; people can return to work; and surgery can be avoided. Like all spinal procedures, this one should not be done on patients taking blood thinners. Other contraindications include local infection in the low back area, presence of a systemic infection, pregnancy, uncontrolled diabetes, and unchecked glaucoma.

Epidurals are typically performed with fluoroscopy, so the physician can observe opaque structures within the body, to ensure that the needle is placed where it is intended. It must go into the correct level in the low back, as well as in the actual area itself. Structures in the epidural space could impede the medication placement; fluoroscopy can prevent medicine from being injected intravascularly. If a patient has had prior surgery, the anatomy can be very abnormal and fluoroscopy can help the practitioner navigate around the changes.

Fluoroscopy does, however, have some shortcomings: expense, short exposure to radiation, and contact with a contrast medium (the dye), which is an allergen for some. If the patient's kidneys do not function properly, dye may cause more damage. Without fluoroscopy, however, there is a 25 percent chance that the medicine will not get to the desired spot.

If after the first injection there is complete resolution of symptoms with accompanying cessation of the use of analgesics and restoration of function, then no other infusions are needed. Treatment can be repeated in the future on an as-needed basis. If there is a partial reduction of symptoms, with a continued need for analgesics, then a repeat injection should be considered. If there is no response to the local anesthetic or steroid, then a nerve root injection can be considered instead. If neither an epidural nor a nerve root injection gives any relief, epidural injections should be discontinued. In my professional opinion only three steroid injections every six months should be undertaken; again, insurance may cover only three in one year.

Typically, people lie prone for a fluoroscopically guided epidural steroid injection. Most physicians do not sedate their patients for this procedure. Monitors such as an EKG, blood pressure, or pulse oximetry are applied. The back is sterilely prepped. Local anesthetic is placed under the skin in order to decrease the sensation of the longer needle needed to complete this job. As the epidural needle is advanced it should create only pressure. If sensations are radiating into the legs, the patient should inform the physician because this may be the start of an avoidable complication. Once the needle is successfully inserted into the epidural space, medicine is injected. The procedure will last approximately two to three minutes from the point the needle first touches the skin. The epidural space can be entered through the center of the back, the lumbar or caudal, or through side openings in the spinal column. Although epidural injections that are done through side openings in the spinal column have many names—including selective nerve root block epidural injection, transforaminal epidural steroid injection, selective epidural block injection, and periradicular infiltration injection—I prefer to call them *selective nerve root injections* or "snerbs."

Snerbs can be more efficient than the typical epidural injections because the medicine is placed directly on the inflamed nerve root. The results in scientific studies from this approach are even more convincing than those from other traditional epidural techniques. The decision to perform one procedure over another is dictated by whether the precise area causing the pain has been identified. A specific location is best approached initially by selective nerve root injections. When the exact area of pathology is undetermined, a translaminar epidural steroid injection should be used. In this approach, the injection is done through the ligament connecting the lamina in adjacent vertebrae.

Epidural Lysis of Adhesions

Some practitioners use an obscure procedure whose efficacy has not been proven. It involves placing a catheter into the epidural space and injecting medicines that are believed to alter adhesions, or scarring, in an area suspected of causing chronic low back pain. Although some people have reported a good response, the initial scientific results are questionable. My concern is that the process doesn't make sense in the context of what we know about the body. Scar, like gristle in steak, is tough—so tough that you need scissors to cut it in order to remove it. Advocates for this procedure claim chemicals can change the scar, but if a formulation is strong enough to alter a scar, wouldn't it also damage neighboring structures like nerves? There has not yet been sufficient research done about this procedure.

Potential Epidural Complications

Though not common when the epidural is performed by an experienced clinician, some problems can occur. A "wet tap" occurs in 1 percent of all epidurals. A wet tap is when the needle tip traverses the epidural space and pierces the dura where spinal fluid is located, which can lead to a positional headache—a headache when you are standing or sitting but not when lying prone. A wet tap will typically respond to rest, caffeinated fluids, and analgesics over two days. If the headache doesn't resolve, a blood patch can help—an epidural injection in which blood is taken from one part of your body and injected into the epidural space. Blood patches are successful in resolving headaches 95 percent of the time.

An allergic reaction can occur during any procedure. Side effects can vary, with rashes and itching the most common. Death from cardiovascular and respiratory failure is possible, although extremely rare. Patients should be observed for allergic reaction after all injections for a period of time. These reactions typically occur within 30 minutes of injection.

Local anesthetic injected into the wrong space could lead to other problems if the dose is high enough. If medication is inserted into the spinal fluid instead of the epidural space, a patient might be unable to move his or her extremities for several hours. If placed into the vasculature, the heart could stop beating. Spinal cord injury can also occur by direct trauma from a needle. The needle could possibly damage the blood supply to the spinal cord, thereby causing a lower-body stroke secondary to a spinal cord infarct (like a heart attack of the spinal cord). If the steroid is injected into an artery supplying the spinal cord, it could result in an infarcted cord.

An epidural abscess occurs when an infection builds up in the spine. This can cause additional problems, the worst being death or sepsis, which is a systemic infection.

A large abscess could compromise the blood flow to the spinal cord, possibly leading to paraplegia. The most common cause of infection is translocation of bacteria from the skin into the epidural space, but fortunately this problem is rare because of sterile preparation of the skin. An epidural abscess could spread and affect other structures. An infection in the bone, called osteomyelitis, can destabilize the spine. An infection in the structures protecting the spinal cord could lead to meningitis.

Absorbed steroids can affect the nervous system, making the patient anxious, irritable, sedated, euphoric, nauseated, or insomniac. They can suppress the body's production of cortisol, often referred to as the "stress hormone," for up to three weeks. Repeated excessive injections can cause a scarcely seen complication: Cushing's syndrome. People with diabetes may have trouble controlling their glucose for a couple of weeks. Occasionally, fluid can be retained, which can make certain underlying health problems such as heart or kidney failure more difficult to control. The excess fluid and accompanying increase in body weight are short lived and rarely permanent.

So, while epidural injections are very useful in treatment and are helpful to many people, they should not be undertaken without a clear understanding of the potential benefits and the potential complications. Talk with your doctor about what you can expect during the procedure, and what symptoms to be on the lookout for after the procedure.

Spinal Cord Stimulation | Overriding pain signals

Patients who find no relief from surgery and whose pain is primarily neuropathic can turn to spinal cord stimulation, a process that mitigates pain by sending new signals to the nervous system that override the pain messages. Most practitioners advocate exhausting all conservative therapies, including opioids, before considering this treatment.

Once spinal cord stimulation is considered, a psychological screening is required by insurance companies to make sure the patient is mentally suited for it. On average, 95 percent of people sent for this testing will be cleared on the first round. After approval for treatment, the patient receives a temporary lead in the back that simulates the permanent device permitting him or her to try out the system. This lead is typically inserted through a needle (it's that small) in an outpatient setting, with no incisions. The goal of spinal cord stimulation is to cause paresthesias (electrical stimulation) in the area of pain without discomfort or muscle contractions.

The procedure to insert the lead does not take long, usually about 15 minutes. The trial lead is kept in place for about a week, which is enough time to assess a patient's response to stimulation. The goal is to cause stimulation during everyday activities to determine if the method will reduce pain and the patient will tolerate the pulses. The trial period is also useful in assessing whether the patient can decrease the use of medications. Once a trial is completed successfully, an outpatient surgical procedure is done to insert the permanent system. If a patient realizes a 50 percent reduction in pain with corresponding improvements in function and reduction in use of oral analgesics, then a permanent spinal cord system can be implanted with confidence. It is installed in the operating room, with the generator implanted into the body. In some systems a receiver is placed under the skin and the power source is externally provided.

Any surgical intervention is associated with a 5 percent chance of infection, which could be as simple as a skin rash but as severe as a rare, but potentially deadly, epidural abscess. Skin problems usually respond to antibiotics, but deeper infections generally require removing the system. The most common complication is lead migration, where the system dislodges and moves. Ten percent of people receiving the system must have it surgically adjusted at some point.

Intrathecal Pumps | Delivering medicine directly

When oral and transdermal opioid and adjunctive therapies are not providing adequate pain relief, intrathecal pumps may be considered. These pumps put medicine directly into the intrathecal space, the fluid surrounding the spinal cord. At Washington University School of Medicine, we generally do not put an intrathecal pump in a person's body for low back pain unless he or she is bedridden and we have tried every other therapeutic option. Most physicians consider the intrathecal pump as the last therapy to try, but some physicians turn to this option sooner. Just as with spinal cord stimulation, with the intrathecal pump, the patient must undergo a psychological assessment before the procedure to implant the pump is done. A patient who is not psychologically fit for the procedure, or who has a clotting disorder, systemic infection, or obstruction of spinal fluid flow should not have an intrathecal pump.

The patient has a trial period of using this device. It is noteworthy that trials vary widely in their performance. For a trial, a catheter is placed in the epidural or intrathecal space in an office or hospital setting and then kept in place for one to seven days. The shorter the trial, the greater the chance of overestimating the benefits of this therapy. But here again, continuing the trial for more than seven days may increase the risk of infection.

If the trial indicates that a patient will benefit from intrathecal medications, a permanent catheter and device are implanted in the operating room. Morphine and baclofen are the only FDA-approved medications for intraspinal infusion, but the list of drugs that can be infused is extensive and includes other opioids, local anesthetics, alpha-adrenoceptor agonists, and novel therapeutics. Use of this device is accepted practice for people with cancer, but it is not generally accepted for treatment of people with chronic low back pain, in part because large-scale studies have yet to be performed. The promise of this technology lies in the variety of drugs that could some day be infused. Identifying the right medication for each patient with the pump is the challenge.

When none of the treatment options discussed so far is effective in reducing your pain to a manageable level, or when your problem might pose a significant risk of permanently damaging your nervous system and therefore affecting your ability to function, surgery may then become a realistic and sometimes necessary intervention.

Chapter 9
Surgery

A treatment of last resort, surgery alters the anatomy to reduce pain.

Note: The anatomy of the back and many of the technical terms used in this chapter are described and illustrated in the appendix. You may want to familiarize yourself with the appendix before reading this chapter.

SPINE SURGERY TECHNIQUES HAVE greatly improved over the past twenty years, and further advances are sure to be made in the coming years. Improved surgical techniques and new technologies make spine surgery a better option than it has been in the past. It is difficult to assess the effectiveness of spine surgery in relation to other treatment approaches, however, because it is not possible to evaluate this surgery in a randomized, double-blind, placebo-controlled study, as we do with other treatments. With other treatments, we know that if a therapy is found to be superior to the placebo, the treatment is justified. But patients' conditions differ, and surgical skills differ, and many other factors differ, so there can be no direct comparison of outcomes for patients who have surgery and those who do not. For this reason, physicians and patients need to give careful consideration before pursuing the surgical option for treating back pain.

Nevertheless, there are situations in which surgery is not just an option—it is an imperative. Any change in neurologic function, such as evolving weakness, loss of sensation, or loss of control of the bowel or bladder, is a sign of nerve damage, and the patient should immediately be evaluated by a surgeon. When function or sensation is affected, surgery may need to be performed to prevent further damage—and sometimes on an emergency basis. In some rare cases the spinal problem causing these symptoms can be treated without surgery and carefully monitored to see whether the symptoms resolve with time, but this scenario is the exception when neurologic function is involved.

Assuming you have normal neurological function, all conservative interventions for reduction of pain should be exhausted before surgery is pursued. While surgery may lead to a reduction of pain in the short term, it could result in further changes in the spine and a potential downward spiral in function. In addition, there are known complication rates with surgery, including the potential for infection and paralysis. You should exhaust every other avenue of treatment first; you should try physical therapy, steroid injections, and months of aggressive medication trials before having surgery.

The cause of most back problems is degeneration, which is the deterioration of cells, tissues, or organs. The end result of degeneration may be a herniated disc or overgrowth of bone. Typically, surgery requires cutting away some tissue and/or fusing one structure to another structure (a procedure called *fusion*) in order to prevent further compromising the spinal cord and avoid nerve damage.

In back surgery, imaging is essential. The surgeon will need to correlate radiographic findings from x-ray, MRI, and so on to the patient's symptoms. Sometimes the plan for surgery is obvious, based on imaging studies and symptoms, but often some uncertainty remains. That is, surgeons operate on the structures in the back that seem to be causing pain or other symptoms, but it may be that the cause of the symptoms is in a different structure. It is not possible always to be accurate about the source of the pain—because of referred pain, for example, which causes symptoms in an area unrelated to the structure that is causing the pain. Through surgery, a surgeon can make the anatomy appear normal, but that doesn't necessarily mean that the pain will go away. If a patient does not have any evidence of nerve damage (as described above), then surgery becomes a form of pain management, albeit an aggressive answer to a problem in the back. Many patients will do extremely well; others may not be as fortunate.

Decompression | Relieving the pressure on discs

Degenerative changes can lead to a disc herniation, also called a ruptured disc. Even without deterioration in the back, occasionally there has been sufficient stress to the disc to cause it to protrude. The disc can exert a mechanical stress on nearby nerves that extend away from the spinal cord, and the patient feels pain in the back and leg. In a discectomy, the disc perceived to be related to the symptoms is excised (cut away) and the nerve is mobilized, that is, freed from surrounding scar tissue. Usually, part of the spinal column is resected (again, cut away) so the surgeon can visualize the disc. Some discectomies can be performed without extracting any of the spinal column, but more typically the disc herniation has occurred laterally (on the side) and requires some removal of spinal bone.

Owing to degenerative changes caused by aging in the spine, discs may protrude, and bone as well as ligament may grow outward, resulting in a gradual compression of the nerves. This condition can occur in the spinal canal, in which case it is known as *spinal stenosis*, or in the canals through which nerves escape the spine, referred to as *spinal foraminal stenosis*. After the neural structures have been compressed, usually gradually and over many years, the symptoms often become noticeable when the person is physically active. For example, the person may feel pain after walking only a few feet, a condition known as *neurogenic claudication*. Early in the disease these stressful occasions will resolve with rest, but as the problem continues over time, pain may occur even during relaxation periods. In lumbar decompressions, the bone perceived to be related to the presenting symptoms is resected. In spinal stenosis, the lamina at one or more levels may be surgically removed. In foraminal stenosis, part of the articular processes may be excised. The earlier the warning signs are addressed, the more likely it is that surgery will be successful.

Fusion | Combining two bones into one

Fusion is the fixation of one bony structure to another; it is an attempt to get two structures to grow together and "fuse" into one. Fusion is based on the theory that if you prevent a painful motion in the spine, the pain should disappear. The best fusing substance is the patient's own bone, although sometimes bone from a donor is used. Recently, modified bone-enhancing protein has also been used for fusion. Regardless of whether the patient's own bone or donor bone is used, a scaffold-like metal structure called *instrumentation* is implanted to help stabilize fused bone while it grows and solidifies in the intended area.

A fusion is typically performed when it is necessary to immobilize a back structure that is unstable and is moving in a way that contributes to back or leg symptoms. Spondylolysis and spondylolisthesis are two conditions that are often treated with fusion. *Spondylolysis* is when a fracture occurs in the pedicles (two small rounded projections from the vertebra—see the appendix), usually at level L5; such a fracture can happen during a traumatic event like a car accident or while performing sports like gymnastics. *Spondylolisthesis* refers to the misalignment of one vertebra in relation to another.

Bones are also fused after a degenerative joint is surgically removed, as is often done in treating spondylosis and scoliosis. In the last ten to fifteen years, vertebral bodies have been increasingly fused together in order to immobilize a disc area believed to contribute to low back pain. Fusion occurs either anteriorly, between vertebral bodies, or posteriorly, between the transverse bodies. Some patients will need both kinds of fusion, or "circumferential" fusion.

There are two types of success in fusion surgery: physical and functional. Physical success is completion of the anatomic changes, as intended, with the bones in alignment and fusion evident. Functional success lies in reduced pain and restored performance. These two achievements do not always correlate, so that while a surgeon may believe that a surgery was well done because the preexisting structural problem was addressed, the patient may not agree if discomfort and impaired mobility continue.

Success rates for fusion vary. In patients with well-defined pathologies like spondylolisthesis or spondylolysis, the outcomes are excellent. In patients where the reasons for the instability and pain are not as clearly defined, the results are not as good.

Disc Replacement | Getting a new disc

A newer therapy for painful lumbar discs is disc replacement. Fusions can immobilize a painful disc and therefore reduce accompanying pain. But immobility in a spinal segment will lead to more rapid degeneration in neighboring spinal segments. A disc replacement alters the painful disc and permits functional mobility to be retained.

Disc replacements do not correct neural compromise, so it is important to have a proper diagnostic workup before pursuing this treatment. The patient's expectations are important in surgery: if you expect an outcome after surgery that the surgery can't possibly accomplish, you will almost certainly be disappointed, and possibly distressed. An MRI or myelogram will help verify that there is no neural compression in the spinal or foraminal canal. A discogram will help clarify which is the painful disc site. These steps will either help you and the surgeon feel more confident that the surgery will bring you relief or they will rule out the surgery as a reasonable approach for treating your condition.

There are many different types of implants. The Link SB and Charité III are the most popular. They are composed of two cobalt-chrome endplates with teeth attached to the vertebral endplates; they also have a sliding polyethylene core. In a disc replacement, the teeth on the endplate for one vertebra connect to the teeth on the endplate for the adjacent vertebra. The purpose of the core is to maintain the mobility of the spine.

Postoperative recovery from disc surgery is typically shorter than from a fusion procedure. Patients are encouraged to progressively mobilize their spine and work toward recovery. This procedure has been performed much longer in Europe than in the United States. There have been no published, prospective, randomized studies comparing disc replacement to fusion.

Spinal Reconstruction | Reshaping the spine

Disruption of the structural integrity of the spine can lead to deformities and instabilities in that area. The causes of this kind of disruption include infection, trauma, tumor, scoliosis (curvature of the spine from side to side, in an S shape), and kyphosis (curvature of the spine resulting in a bowing of the back). Another possible cause is a surgery in which too much bone was resected, resulting in structural instability. Surgical correction of deformities and instabilities in the spine involves altering tissues to permit realignment and fusion, with the goal of preventing recurrence. Various forms of metal support may be used as a type of scaffolding in order to permit bone to fuse.

With the aging of our society, more spinal deformities will occur and therefore more spinal reconstruction will take place. Just as with other surgical procedures, if you have normal neurological function, you should exhaust all nonsurgical treatments before pursuing surgery.

Chapter 10
Alternative Treatments

Complementary medicine is evolving. Experiment and discover its possible benefits.

WHAT IF YOU'VE ADOPTED many of the techniques discussed in previous chapters but you still feel that something's missing? Maybe you've changed your diet, restructured your work to allow for more rest periods, added a comfortable exercise regimen, and become an optimist—but you still need to alleviate your pain. Alternative therapies are available that can complement the approaches discussed in previous chapters.

In alternative or complementary medicine, the mental and emotional aspects of healing are intertwined with the physical. Maintaining a healthy balance is essential to success with these kinds of therapy, which include acupuncture, acupressure, biofeedback, herbal medication, magnetic therapy, bodywork (through Pilates or yoga, therapeutic massage, Rolfing, and therapeutic touch), and prayer. You may want to experiment. Find out if one (or more) of these approaches works for you and add it to the traditional methods offered by your physician.

In choosing an alternative medicine practitioner, use many of the same criteria you would to choose a physician. You will want to find someone with whom you have good rapport. A referral from either a trusted friend or your doctor is a good place to start. Ask about that person's bedside manner, philosophy, and practices. You will want the professional to be

sensitive to your goals and expectations. Since chronic low back pain requires a multidisciplinary approach, you should avoid anyone who refuses
to work with your physician.

Most doctors are happy to discuss the appropriate use of complementary
and alternative therapies. If your doctor does not want you to participate
in alternative therapies, you may want to re-evaluate whether he or she
shares your views. Your physician may not agree with all contemporary
therapies, but it is his or her responsibility to explain them to you. Ask
your doctor whether, given your health, condition, and circumstances,
there are any potential risks to using contemporary therapies. Some people should avoid certain therapies. Your doctor can advise you best.

Acupuncture and Acupressure | Ancient Chinese techniques

Acupuncture, practiced in China for more than 5,000 years, is one of the
most commonly used alternative medicine approaches in the treatment of
back pain. Today, thousands of physicians practice acupuncture to treat
chronic pain. In traditional Chinese medicine, the human body is considered a miniature model of the universe; therefore the rules that govern
the universe also regulate the body.

The main principles at the foundation of acupuncture are the yin-yang
and the Five Elements. The yin-yang is based on the idea of duality;
an imbalance of this duality leads to illnesses. The Five Elements—fire,
earth, metal, water, and wood—are believed to have a regulatory effect
on one another and cannot exist without each other.

The energy that flows through this Eastern system is called the "qi,"
which is thought of as the vital life energy present in all things. Qi, also
called chi, circulates in the body along twelve to fourteen energy pathways called meridians. The meridians are located on each side of the body
and cross along the arms, legs, torso, and head. Each meridian is thought
to be linked with a specific internal organ or organ system. The meridian
rises to the surface at different locations on the body, and this is where
the acupuncture points are located. When stimulated, these points cause
healing to take place. Special needles are placed just under the surface of
the skin at specific acupoints, providing the right amount of stimulation
to correct and redirect the balance of energy flow. The opposing forces,

known within the body as the yin and the yang, must be in balance before the qi can help the spiritual, mental, physical, and emotional components to resume working normally.

Acupuncture is an acceptable alternative therapy that can be included in a comprehensive treatment plan. As with any office visit, a trip to the acupuncturist should start with a detailed history and a physical examination tailored to your pain state. It's important to inform your acupuncturist about any medications—both prescription and herbal—that you're taking, to prevent any life-threatening complication.

Your practitioner may examine your tongue, which is considered to be the primary source of diagnostic information, and record additional information about body language, the color of your urine, sensitivity to temperatures and seasons, and eating and sleeping habits. Some of this may seem strange to patients accustomed to Western medical practices, but unfamiliar alternative medicine should be approached with an open mind.

After completing the examination, the acupuncturist will place special needles in appropriate acupoints. The needles are very thin, ranging from 1/17,000 to 1/18,000 of an inch in diameter. They are traditionally made of stainless steel with copper overlay, but can also be silver, bamboo, or wood. Be sure your acupuncturist uses needles that are sterile and disposable. Depending upon the pain, anywhere from ten to twelve needles may be placed at particular locations. They are meant to remove blockages in the meridian and improve the flow of the qi. You'll notice, no doubt, that the needle placement doesn't seem to correlate with the location of your pain symptoms. That's because they are placed on meridian points. After the needles are placed, the acupuncturist may twist them in a circular motion for 15 to 20 seconds and leave them in for approximately 15 to 30 minutes, after which they're removed and you can resume activities.

Adverse effects with acupuncture are minimal and rare but can include infection, bleeding, and collapsed lung—a condition known as pneumothorax. Common side effects reported in patients undergoing acupuncture include sleepiness, fatigue, bruising, dizziness, and increased severity of pain upon insertion of the needle.

Acupuncture can be highly effective when used in combination with a comprehensive treatment program, but just how effective acupuncture is continues to be controversial. Although many patients report that acupuncture changes their perception of pain, there are few scientific studies demonstrating its effectiveness. In 1998, a panel of experts from the National Institutes of Health concluded that acupuncture was effective in two conditions: helping to resolve postoperative pain and chemotherapy-induced nausea. The panel further concluded that acupuncture could be effective in other conditions, such as low back pain, headaches, and fibro-myalgia, but that further research was needed.[1]

Acupressure stems from the same Chinese belief that restoring the flow of the qi will relieve symptoms of pain and illness. During acupressure, the practitioner applies pressure with his or her fingers to specific points of the body. There are no needles involved. The pressure improves the flow of qi and decreases pain.

Biofeedback | Relax and listen to your body

Biofeedback uses technology to teach you how your body responds, with the goal of reducing pain. During a biofeedback session, a therapist will apply electrodes to various parts of your body. The electrodes are then attached to a monitoring device that provides feedback on what your body is doing.

This information includes brain wave activity, breathing, heart rate, blood pressure, and muscle tension. With the electrodes in place, the therapist will use relaxation techniques to calm you, reducing your muscle tension and decreasing your heart rate and blood pressure. The goal is for you to enter into a relaxed state, thus improving your coping skills. You watch the monitor to get "feedback" on how your body is responding to the therapist's efforts. Eventually you will learn to relax consciously on your own, without the need for instruction from the therapist or feedback from the monitor. Biofeedback is traditionally performed by psychologists and physical therapists.

Herbal Medication | Nature's medicine

Before the advent of modern medicine, many practitioners used various herbs and plants to treat common ailments. An estimated 250,000 to 500,000 plants exist in the world today, and approximately 25 percent of all prescription medication is derived from trees, plants, or herbs. Herbs can be consumed in teas, capsules, tablets, tinctures, and essential oils; they can also be applied to the skin in salves and ointments.

Incorporating herbal medications into your treatment plan can be as simple as researching them and choosing one that appeals to you. You can purchase herbal medications over the counter (without a prescription). A more systematic approach would involve consulting a Chinese medicine practitioner. These herbalists follow a philosophy not rooted in traditional Western beliefs. In treating back pain, they rely on the use of herbs, exercises, and acupuncture. An Ayurvedic, another type of herbal practitioner, uses the connection of mind, body, and spirit to treat pain. These practitioners may also incorporate diet, herbs, relaxation techniques, massage, and exercise.

When deciding whether to use herbal medications, keep in mind that a product advertised as "all natural" does not necessarily imply safe. Unlike prescription medications, which undergo years of clinical research and ultimate approval by the U.S. Food and Drug Administration before they are made available to patients, herbal medications are not regulated by any medical body and therefore have little or no clinical research to back their claims. If you use herbal medications, be cautious. Never exceed the recommended dosing schedule. You should also examine the interactions, potency, form, cultivation, containments, and added ingredients of herbals. Consult your physician before taking any herbals because some of them should not be taken with certain prescription medications, as interactions have occurred.

Selecting the Right Herbs in Small Doses

Because herbal medicine is not regulated, the same herbal medication can vary from brand to brand in its potency and recommended doses. When introducing one of these herbals, it's a good idea to start with a small dose and then, as you tolerate it, gradually increase until you achieve the desired effect. You can take some of the guesswork out of herbals by seeking out preparations that are "standardized," which means they meet an international standard of quality.

Not all herbals are made with products grown in the United States. Some may be cultivated in South America or other regions of the world where insecticides and pesticides not necessarily permitted in our country

are used, or where contamination by arsenic, mercury, and lead has occurred. You should be careful to purchase herbal medication that has
been produced and packaged according to strict quality control measures.
Occasionally herbal medications include other ingredients that may not
be listed on the bottle and may interact with prescription medications.
That's why the rule of thumb is always to check with your physician.

Herbs Used to Treat Low Back Pain

Boswellia, a commonly used herb, has been studied as an alternative to
aspirin. It is thought to have an anti–inflammatory mediator that inhibits
leukotrienes, part of the immune system that contributes to inflammation. Taking this herb may decrease joint inflammation and swelling and
increase mobility. Side effects can include gastrointestinal discomfort.

Capsicum, an herb found in chili peppers, Tabasco, and paprika, can
be a potent pain reliever when applied directly to the skin. Capsicum
works by reducing substance P, a neuropeptide that carries pain signals
throughout the body. A skin test should be performed to check for potential sensitivities; contact with eyes or open wounds can cause a burning
sensation; and if taken in large doses, stomach upset and diarrhea can
result.

Feverfew works by decreasing prostaglandin levels, which results in
reduced pain and inflammation. Feverfew can be taken as a powder or
a tablet and is relatively safe except in individuals taking blood thinners,
such as Coumadin or Plavix.

Two over-the-counter dietary substances have been shown to decrease
pain: glucosamine and chondroitin. These are naturally occurring amino
sugars found in joints and connective tissue responsible for maintaining
the lubrication of the joint and slowing the breakdown of cartilage. As
with any herbal or dietary supplement, glucosamine and chondroitin are
unregulated and their potency and quality will vary from brand to brand.
Glucosamine comes from shellfish, so anyone with an allergy to shellfish
should avoid it. Traditionally, it takes two to four weeks for any noticeable benefit to be realized from either of these two substances.

Magnetic Therapy | Placing magnets on the skin

Magnetic therapy involves exposing parts of the body to a magnetic field, thus stimulating the body's natural electrical field. This therapy can be used on a small scale with magnets, usually in the form of bracelets, applied to the skin, or it can involve higher levels of magnetism when applied on a large scale. Magnetic therapy for chronic back pain involves placing magnets at tender points on the back.

The basic premise is that the magnets have two poles: a positive and a negative. The negative pole emits a calming, healing effect, whereas the positive pole is associated with stress. Prolonged exposure to the latter can be ultimately unhealthy. The strength of a magnet is measured in units of gauss; the amount of gauss decreases with distance from the body.

While no clinical scientific evidence exists regarding the effectiveness of magnetic therapy, there are many who believe in its power. Theories on how magnet therapy works rely on the notion that magnets help increase blood flow to the tender areas on the body. Increased blood flow carries more oxygen, which in turn decreases inflammation and relieves pain. Another theory suggests that a magnetic field disrupts the pain signal going to the brain, thereby allowing the release of endorphins, the body's natural pain-killing substance, from the brain.

Despite the lack of clinical studies evaluating the safety and efficacy of magnetic therapy, there are no documented serious side effects. As with any alternative therapy, getting clearance from your physician is essential. If you wear an implantable device, such as a pacemaker, inform your doctor first and do not place a magnet directly over the device, because doing so could cause complications. It is never a good idea to use this therapy during pregnancy, and you should avoid using a magnetic bed for longer than eight to ten hours at a time.

Bodywork | Move your body

Bodywork refers to therapies that include massage, deep tissue manipulation, energy balancing, and movement awareness. When used correctly, bodywork can reduce pain, stimulate blood and lymphatic circulation, promote relaxation, and relieve injured muscles. Traditional bodywork treatment includes four common elements: pressure to alter the muscles and tissues; patient education about and awareness of how posture and movement affect physical functioning and reduce pain; stretching and relaxation; and breathing and stress management techniques to decrease tension and enhance overall well-being.

Pilates

Pilates is a system developed by Joseph Pilates that focuses on physical conditioning with a strong emphasis on proper body alignment, prevention of further injury, and correct breathing techniques. It also incorporates muscle stretching and strengthening. The goal of Pilates is to encourage a lengthening of the muscles. It promotes body balance and stabilization of the spine.

Depending upon your unique needs, you might simply take advantage of Pilates floor exercises, or you might use Pilates equipment with springs and ropes for added resistance. You may be asked to lie, sit, stand, or kneel on a movable bench while at the same time pushing or pulling with your feet and hands, utilizing a strap, bar, or pulley.

In Pilates, the abdominal muscles are the main focal point of each movement, along with concentration on proper breathing, ease of motion, and relaxation. To do Pilates safely, you must work with a certified Pilates professional.

Yoga

Yoga is an ancient form of exercise shown to reduce stress, increase range of motion, and improve strength. Posture yoga alleviates typical aches and strains, while concentration yoga assists in overcoming the mental component of pain. Meditation exercises help people put their condition into context and refocus breathing to decrease their level of discomfort. See chapter 5 for a more complete discussion of the benefits of yoga.

Therapeutic Massage

Massage is one of the most commonly used hands-on approaches for treating musculoskeletal pain. Research indicates that massage therapy significantly decreased pain in the patients surveyed. In addition to providing relief, therapeutic massage improved circulation and joint mobility and reduced muscle tension.

Massage therapy activates the body's release of endorphins, serotonin, and norepinephrine, all substances that relieve pain. It also increases circulation by decreasing swelling and moving the excess fluid into the circulatory system. Muscle tension, regardless of its cause—whether injury, activity, or stress—can result in muscle fatigue. Contraction of the muscles for a prolonged period of time leads to tissue destruction by interfering with the elimination of chemical waste products. The longer a muscle is tense, the more waste builds up; eventually the nerve becomes irritated, and then the discomfort gets worse. Massage loosens tight, overstressed muscles, decreasing the tension that can cause spasms, and improves joint mobility by enhancing blood flow to the affected areas.

There are different kinds of massages available; find the one that best suits your needs.

Deep tissue massage uses slow strokes and deep finger pressure to break the cycle of muscle tension. Its focus is on the deeper layers of tissue, the tendons.

Swedish massage is based on a system that uses long strokes, friction, and kneading on the top layers of the muscle. The therapist utilizes both passive and active range of motion. Kneading of the muscles involves squeezing and rolling.

Chair massage is done while the client is fully clothed and seated in a specially designed chair that allows the therapist to have full access to the client's back. A chair massage session may last between 15 and 60 minutes. Its purpose is to promote relaxation and improve circulation.

Reflexology is massage based on a system of "points" on the feet and hands that "reflex back" to different areas of the body. Massaging a certain area of the hand, for example, can relieve a body part such as a painful low back.

Rolfing

Rolfing, developed by Dr. Ida Rolf in 1970, relies on the notion that the body structures affect all physical and psychological processes. It is based on the idea that human functioning improves only when the body is properly balanced. Dr. Rolf believed that when the body is out of alignment, the muscles become contracted and other tissues in the body then have to compensate, causing further stress to the body. Movement is impaired and a cascade of events follows, including increased emotional stress and decreased mental clarity.

When Rolfing is performed, the practitioner seeks to re-establish the body's balance by performing a series of manipulations that apply pressure to the fascia—a thin, elastic membrane that encases every muscle, bone, blood vessel, nerve, and organ in the body. The pressure, which can be brought about with the practitioner's fingers, knuckles, or elbow, can cause mild to severe discomfort. It is through these manipulations, however, that pain relief is theoretically achieved.

Therapeutic Touch

Therapeutic touch was first developed by a nurse, Dolores Krieger, a professor at New York University. This technique harkens back to the concept of "laying on of hands," in which restorative power was believed to flow from the faith healer to the sick person. The term "therapeutic touch" is a bit of a misnomer here, because the therapist does not actually place his or her hands on the patient; rather, the practitioner simulates the necessary movement. Therapeutic touch derives from the notions that the body generates a field of energy and that a disruption in this field can cause disease and illness. Consequently, practitioners try to rid the patient of any imbalance by moving their hands back and forth across the area, to encourage healing and reduce pain through a transfer of energy.

Prayer | For those who believe

Although many people would not consider prayer a form of alternative medicine, it is widely accepted as just that. In fact, it is thought to be the most common wellness-related practice in the United States. In 1988, a poll of approximately 2,000 people found that 35 percent used prayer for health-related concerns.[2] An additional 22 percent stated that they prayed about specific medical conditions, and approximately 66 percent said they believed that prayer was very helpful to them. Prayer is related to the concept of a mind-body connection that maintains that healing the mind will heal the body as well. Prayer has no known negative effects and should be pursued by individuals who believe in its healing power.

Part of my education has involved the study of religion at Yale University's Divinity School. I have seen that belief can be very powerful and motivational for behavior. Acting on belief through prayer can change an individual, which may manifest itself by better health as well as better management of chronic pain.

Part III

The Cost of Chronic Pain

Chapter 11
Covering the Cost of Pain
❧ *Insurance*

Insurance companies influence health care decisions.

HEALTH CARE IN AMERICA teaches us a different golden rule—those with the gold make the rules. That's why insurance carriers dictate much of the health care in this country. First you have to pay high premiums to get them to cover you. Then doctors are always butting heads with them over the appropriate care for patients. Finally, the best therapies must often be sacrificed in favor of the least expensive approach.

It is estimated that back pain costs the United States up to $100 billion each year through lost work days and reduced productivity. In this country, back problems are the most frequently filed workers' compensation disability claims in individuals under 45 years of age.

Insurance Plans | HMOs, PPOs, and Medicare

When it comes to health care insurance in the United States, people usually have the choice between two business models: managed care or a fee-for-service plan. Managed care offers general coverage but limits the possible avenues of treatment; it is known as an HMO, or health maintenance organization. Fee-for-service insurance is more expensive for the patient, because the insurance typically pays 80 percent of the medical charges and the patient covers the remaining 20 percent. This format is known as a PPO, or preferred provider organization. Few people can afford this system.

Typically HMOs operate through a primary care physician who first assesses your problem. Your doctor can refer you to a specialist when your situation falls outside his or her area of expertise. When it is appropriate your doctor may order tests, but often the tests can be done only after the HMO has approved the order.

PPOs offer special services to member organizations that have contracted with them for care. As an individual, if you select this system you may pay slightly higher rates and expect more than from an HMO. Usually you can choose from a larger group of doctors and you may use a specialist outside your coverage if you're willing to pay more in your co-pay.

Medicare covers people over age 65 and disabled people. It has three parts: part A covers facility fees; part B, professional services; and part D, prescription medications. Private companies have contracted to administer part D, which has led to much confusion. There are too many choices with too little clarity. Very few patients have mastered the intricacies of part D, and many physicians have been thwarted by the system as well. That's because medications that have been working for a patient can be summarily changed, depending upon who is administering part D. For example, you may be stable on daily OxyContin 80 mg, but the new administrators of your prescriptions may question whether you still need to be on this medication. If the physician justifies the treatment, the carrier may still want proof that you wouldn't benefit from other, less expensive medications, such as methadone or morphine. The back and forth negotiations can lead to periods of uncertainty and a loss of progress in pain management.

Medication | Sources and considerations

Medication costs cause stress and undue hardship for many people. Some people do without necessities like food and heat to obtain medicine; others shortchange their treatments because they can't afford to take all the recommended medications. Because markup on pharmaceuticals can vary substantially, a growing number of people are turning to foreign countries to obtain medicine at less expensive prices.

The Internet provides access to many medications, which isn't always a good thing. Be sure that any company you deal with is a United States company, because then you know its products are regulated by federal oversight through the Food and Drug Administration (FDA). Even drugs from Canada can be suspect. Drug manufacturers in Canada may take the active agent and add other chemicals—such as additives to make the pill stick together, or colors, and so on. These additional chemicals may not be permissible in our country and, in some instances, could even be deemed dangerous by our regulators. Also, never buy narcotics via the Internet. There is no control over these narcotics on the Internet, and if you are enrolled in a pain management program, you may be violating agreements about your care with your treating physician.

Insurance companies create lists, called *formularies,* of the medications they will cover. Some medications—generally the ones that cost more—are better than others. Many insurance companies will only pay for generic drugs when a generic version is available; the generic is almost always cheaper than the brand drug. The generics can be as effective as the big brands, but these formularies limit physicians' choices and can prevent them from providing the medication they deem best to address your situation. For example, many pain physicians, myself included, advocate sustained-release opioids so that patients don't have to take medications as frequently. The insurance company, however, may try to substitute with methadone because it is the cheapest narcotic available to treat chronic pain.

I have seen that methadone has many side effects; it is generally considered the most difficult opioid to use. Usually, methadone has to be taken several times a day, which decreases compliance, and converting from any narcotic to methadone is challenging, because the pharmacology of the drug can vary greatly in individuals, making it easier to overdose.

We can't know at this point what government health care plans and private insurance plans will look like in the future. A national health care plan may make it easier for some people to gain access to health care and medications, especially people who currently have difficulty getting health care and paying for medications. It may also make it more expensive if not more difficult for others to do so.

For the time being, the best advice is to work with your physician and your health care insurance provider, or Medicare, to make decisions based on your symptoms, your doctor's findings, and the results of diagnostic tests.

Chapter 12
The Ins and Outs of Disability

Navigating through a sea of regulations and applications is daunting but doable.

MOST OF THE PATIENTS I see at the pain management center want to continue working and are seeking ways to return to their current jobs, even when they are faced with major physical challenges. However, there are situations when the effects of an injury or illness become so debilitating that the person can no longer function in a work environment. When this happens, the issue of disability benefits arises.

Although there may be numerous disability benefit programs available to an individual, the two most significant categories are the government plans administered under the Social Security Administration and private short-term and long-term disability insurance plans available to individuals either through their workplace or by individual purchase, independent of employment.

Social Security Disability | The government's plans

There are two disability programs under Social Security Administration control: SSDI (Social Security Disability Insurance benefits) and SSI (disability-based Supplemental Security Income). Each of the Administration's programs has at its core the issue of whether the applicant is "disabled" for the purposes of Social Security. The Administration has certain thresholds that must be met at each level of its inquiry as it also considers alternatives to a disability finding. Only when an individual meets all the necessary criteria will the Administration enter a determination that the applicant is disabled and is entitled to benefits. At any level, should the applicant not meet the threshold criteria, or should an alternative be lawfully available, the Administration may deny the application and benefits.

Disability insurance benefits (SSDI) are employment-based, determined by the applicant's earnings and years of productivity. An applicant for disability insurance benefits must have worked in positions where Social Security taxes (FICA) were deducted from his or her income and must have accumulated sufficient credits during employment to be eligible. Because the amount of credits available to a given individual adjusts annually, it is important to refer to the literature provided by the Social Security Administration concerning eligibility. Should an applicant have sufficient credits, then he or she will be deemed eligible for disability insurance benefits.

Supplemental Security Income (SSI) is determined by the financial need of the applicant, based upon specific criteria. It is limited to individuals whose income and assets fall below specified levels. These levels change, so, again, an applicant should refer to the literature provided by the Social Security Administration. Once an applicant is accepted into a need-based program, that need must continue. Should an applicant's assets or income exceed those permitted under the program, his or her benefits will be terminated.

Under both Social Security disability programs, you as the claimant must be incapable of working at your present job owing to your impairment. Further, if under the age of 52, you must be unable to execute any other occupation that you performed in the past and must also be deemed unfit to be trained to fill a new position.

Short-Term and Long-Term Disability Benefits | Private plans

Short- and long-term disability programs are independent from Social Security benefits. These private plans can be purchased through the workplace or by an individual, and they afford coverage to the policyholder should he or she become disabled during the period of time specified in the contract. Policies differ as to the amount of benefit paid, the length of coverage, exclusions, and, most importantly, the provision for ongoing care, as well as the basis for termination of benefits.

Short-term disability is exactly what it says—it is a disability benefit available for a short period of time. When a covered individual becomes incapable of performing the duties of his or her present employment, this policy will provide assistance in the short term. Usually, the time from the onset of the disabling condition to the end of the recovery period must fall between a minimum of one week to a maximum of one year; however, in some policies these limits are less well defined.

Long-term disability is intended for individuals whose condition will make it impossible to perform the present job-related duties for the foreseeable future. In addition, most long-term disability contracts require that the claimant be unable to work at any other employment that may be available, either through the claimant's experience or capabilities or through retraining. Finally, long-term disability contracts generally require that, once approved for payments, the claimant continues to receive ongoing care and treatment from a health care provider for that disability.

Am I Disabled? | If so, what's next?

Disability has many different definitions. Your health care provider will tell you whether, in his or her opinion, your physical or mental condition is such that you are rendered disabled. Generally, a disability is any condition that compromises an individual's ability to perform certain tasks, movements, activities, or functions.

A disability can take many forms, from physical or mechanical in nature that restrict a person's power to move, lift, or act, to emotional elements that limit a person's ability to interact with other people. The condition may be based in an injury, an illness, a genetic disorder, or any combination thereof. The tasks limited by the person's circumstances may be any in a wide range, from the most basic functions, such as walking, lifting, standing, or kneeling, to the most complex, such as an inability to formulate words and phrases or to follow instructions.

Conditions that limit your abilities may be difficult to perceive. The onset or progress may be slow and gradual, such as with a degenerative process like osteoarthritis or multiple sclerosis. It may be chronic in nature, having been present for so long—as in a latent birth defect, for example—that you have unknowingly adapted to its presence (though such condition may worsen over time). At other times, however, the onset may be sudden in nature, resulting from an injury.

When you first realize you have a condition that impedes your ability to act, whether it comes on gradually or acutely, you should make an appointment with your health care provider. Any such circumstances, whether physical or mental in nature, must be quickly and accurately evaluated by your physician. As always, it is vitally important to advise your doctor of all relevant details, including any factors that caused the onset or worsening of your symptoms. Cooperate fully with your health care provider, including having all diagnostic studies that may be ordered to assist in a thorough evaluation of your problem.

Be proactive. Ask your doctor about his or her findings and diagnosis; discuss with your doctor the nature of the condition, its extent, whether it is temporary or permanent in nature, and the various treatment options. Do not be reluctant to inquire about alternative therapies; remember that your doctor is there to assist you. Ask specifically whether this finding renders you disabled in any manner, and how this condition will affect your ability to work. Be prepared to describe in detail the nature of the work you perform, but allow the physician to determine what, if any, new challenges will result from your condition.

Should your doctor decide that a disability is present, he or she may place certain parameters on your activities. These limitations can take many forms, including restrictions on the amount and manner of lifting (for example, no more than 10 pounds, no lifting above the level of the shoulders) and the nature of body movement (for example, no kneeling, bending from the waist, or squatting). Ask whether these restrictions will be permanent, because the duration of the restrictions will enter into any determination regarding a possible disability.

If your doctor prescribes medication, ask about the medicine's intended use, the manner in which it works, its side effects, and what outcome you should expect from the medication. You can also get this information from your pharmacist. Find out how long your doctor anticipates you will be taking the medication and if there are any long-term effects. A medical problem that is significant enough to require medications may be significant enough to warrant disability.

The presence of a disability in and of itself does not preclude continued employment. Many individuals who suffer from a disability are capable of functioning daily in an employment setting as a result of medication, therapy, treatment, accommodation, altered work spaces, or other means of assistance. More than the mere presence of a disability is required in order for an individual to receive aid in the form of benefits, whether paid by a private insurer or by the Social Security Administration.

Once you have seen your physician, consider the parameters placed on your ability to perform tasks that are required in your job. If the restrictions limit you but do not prevent you from performing your duties—if certain reasonable changes are made to accommodate your abilities—then although you are disabled, you may not qualify for disability benefits. However, should your condition prevent you from performing your basic job duties, even with accommodation, then you have met the initial threshold for obtaining disability: the condition you have prevents you from returning to your present employment.

The next question is whether the disability is such that you cannot work at any other employment. Social Security and disability insurance through a private carrier usually approach this issue from different perspectives. Both generally require a comprehensive list of your prior employment in order to determine whether your restrictions, which may prevent you from working at your present job, will permit you to work in any prior position. If so, under Social Security should you be younger than 52, you may be denied benefits; this factor has little impact on the applications of individuals over the age of 52, however. Under private carrier insurance the issue of employability at a prior position is usually relevant for all ages. If you can work at a former job, even taking into account your restrictions, then long-term disability will be denied.

Finally, there is the issue of retraining. Both Social Security, in the case of individuals under the age of 52, and private long-term disability insurers will review your capabilities and restrictions to determine whether, given your age, education, physical and mental capacities, and background, you would be able to be retrained for any other gainful employment in the open job market. If so, then disability will be denied. In some cases Social Security will arrange for the claimant's attendance at a vocational rehabilitation center to assist in this retraining.

The Application Process | Organize, then apply

If you feel that you have met the requisite criteria to apply for benefits—through either Social Security, short- or long-term disability, or both—then it is time to apply. However, first you must organize your information. Create a disability file to store your records and copies of all relevant documents:

- Obtain a copy of your Social Security card and your birth certificate or baptismal record.
- Start a log of the health care providers you've seen regarding any condition that contributes to your disability, noting their names, addresses, specialties, dates of visits, examinations, and treatments.
- Maintain a list of all the medicine you take and its dosage.
- Add copies of any relevant medical records or laboratory results to your file.
- Detail your employment history and educational achievements.
- Include verification of U.S. citizenship or eligible noncitizen status, with a resident alien card issued by the federal government.
- Include a copy of your most recent W-2 form, or, if self-employed, your latest federal tax returns.
- Include a copy of the contract of disability insurance (if seeking disability benefits from a private insurer or employer).

Keep a copy of each application that you submit. File all correspondence received from any party concerning your application, including denial or award letters. Start a calendar of events, noting doctor visits, when letters were received, dates when information was provided, and other important points of time relating to your condition and/or application process.

Under Social Security guidelines, you must contact your local Administration Office and inform them of your desire to apply for disability benefits. In some instances this application can be taken over the telephone or via the Internet. However, to speed the application process and permit the presentation of the documents contained in your file, it is best to file in person.

If applying for SSI, in addition to the documents noted above, you should also be prepared to provide information about the home where you live—which would include lease or rental documents or a copy of a mortgage—as well as your payroll slips, bank books, insurance policies, burial fund records, and other information about your income and possessions.

Short-term and long-term disability, if available through your employer, must be applied for through your human resources department. Again, this application, generally provided by the insurer to your employer, must be completed with accuracy. If you purchased your disability insurance independently, then you must contact the insurance company directly to obtain a claim form—which should be filled out and returned as quickly as possible. It must be noted that applications to the insurance carriers must follow the instructions of the insurance company; applications that are not properly filled out, or not submitted in the manner required, or not filed within the time frame specified, may be denied—even if you are disabled.

For both Social Security and private insurance applications, it is vital that you provide all information requested. This would include all pertinent details regarding your past employment history, your educational background, and the conditions that restrict or preclude your ability to work. It is also important that you supply the names of all health care providers who have treated you for any condition you have listed.

The Need for Records | Physician records are crucial

Both Social Security and disability insurance benefits from a private carrier rely on physicians' findings as contained in the documented records that should be maintained by your health care providers. Although there are provisions for direct testimony by the various doctors, on the whole these claims are awarded or denied based on documents. Without a verifiable diagnosis by a physician showing a debilitating condition that impedes your ability to be gainfully employed—backed by examination results, patient complaints, laboratory reports, and other similar records contained within a medical file—an application for disability benefits will generally be denied.

Thus it is vitally important that your physician fully, completely, and legibly document diagnosis, disability restrictions, examination results, patient complaints, laboratory reports, and other matters related to your case. The purpose of this documentation is twofold. First, it enables subsequent health providers to review, complement, and further your treatment, and to understand the basis for your physician's diagnosis and modality of care. Second, for purposes of disability, it permits the evaluator of your disability application to determine the basis for such diagnosis, and how that diagnosis impacts your ability to function in the workplace. This documentation should include the date of initial examination, the nature of your complaints, objective and subjective findings, diagnosis, and course of treatment. Do not hesitate to ask the physician to fully document your visit or visits and his or her findings.

Your disability claim may result in your being examined by more than one physician. This is not unusual in even the simplest of disabling conditions. For this reason, it is also important for you to maintain an accurate and complete record of your examinations. Include the date and time of the examination or visit, the name of the physician who examined you, and a short note indicating your complaints, the nature of your examination, and what was discussed concerning your condition, including the treatment to be followed. Keep all documents received by you from the physician's office, including receipts, copies of prescriptions, and appointment reminder cards.

Sometimes disability providers may require you to be examined by a physician of their choosing to determine the nature and extent of your disability. Again, this is not unusual, and cooperation with this doctor is encouraged. Once more, thoroughly describe the nature of your condition, including the effects of any medication(s) you are taking.

At times, depending upon the nature of the condition, you may wish to keep a copy of your own medical records. Under the laws of most states you are entitled to this information. Your records should include all notes, laboratory reports, x-rays, and other similar documents. Most states allow the physician to charge a nominal fee for copying these items. While these records, being supplied directly by you without certification, may have less credence than those same records coming directly from the physician's office, should the latter be unavailable for any reason, your submission will at least be viewed as showing that you have a documented condition for which treatment was sought.

Although Social Security will usually obtain the relevant medical records pertaining to your condition, it is a good idea for you to routinely check with your Social Security processor to ensure that progress is being made. Your assistance in obtaining records may be necessary or, due to the volume of cases processed by Social Security, the Administration may overlook records that may be relevant to your claim and you will need to bring these records to their attention.

Likewise, some short-term and long-term disability benefit insurance carriers will obtain the necessary records from your health care provider for their review in determination of your claim. Others will place that responsibility with you. Make sure to check the contract with your insurer to clarify these details. Under all circumstances do as required; failure to cooperate can lead to a denial of your claim, even in the face of a disabling condition.

Finally, note that obtaining disability based solely upon your complaints is generally difficult. Your condition needs to be documented and verified independently by a health care provider. Your unconfirmed testimony before the Social Security Administration has less credibility than qualified testimony supported by competent medical records. Disability benefits from an insurance carrier are based almost solely upon medical records, so documenting the disabling condition through examination by a health care provider, and through medical records, is vital.

The Determination Process | Decisions and appeals

The process of determining whether a person qualifies for disability benefits differs slightly between the government and private programs. Both have an investigative procedure and provide avenues for appeal, but the details of their programs vary, so familiarize yourself with their policies as applicable to your individual circumstances.

The Social Security Administration sometimes utilizes outside agencies to assist in gathering the information necessary to make a determination. It generally takes from three to five months to process a claim for disability benefits. In arriving at its decision, the Administration reviews your statements regarding your abilities, both during the interview process and through a written questionnaire. However, more importantly, the Administration looks at the relevant medical records concerning your physical and mental condition. It takes into consideration the limitations placed on you by examining health care providers and how those restrictions impact your ability to perform tasks necessary to be employable.

Once that determination is made, a letter informing you of the decision is mailed. If their finding is favorable, your file is placed in line for payment. If the decision is unfavorable, you have sixty days from the date of the decision letter to file a request for a hearing before an administrative law judge.

In a hearing, the administrative law judge will take your testimony regarding your limitations and how your condition affects your ability to work. If you are under 52, the judge may also hear testimony from a vocational expert as to whether, given your restrictions, there are any jobs available to you. The administrative law judge may also receive additional evidence in the form of medical records or other documents at this time, and he or she may agree to hold your record open for a period of time, to permit other relevant data to be obtained, if necessary. When the judge makes his or her determination, a letter is sent to you outlining the reason for the decision. If favorable, your file is placed in line for payment. If unfavorable, you may submit an application for review of the judge's decision to the Appeals Council and include further evidence if applicable. If the Appeals Council denies your appeal, you can file a suit before the U.S. District Court.

Applications for short-term and long-term disability to private insurers undergo a similar review initially. Your medical records are examined by an evaluator at the insurance company. They may also be reviewed, at the request of the insurance company, by another health care provider paid by the insurer. The insurance company may also contact the treating physicians to ask if—in their opinion—you have the ability to perform tasks necessary to be employable, as well as the nature and extent of any limitations on your basic movements. At the completion of this review, the insurance company will issue a letter informing you of its decision and of any appeals process permitted under the contract of insurance and federal law.

Following a Favorable Award | Receiving benefits

Should you file for both Social Security and private short-term or long-term insurance disability benefits, and be approved for both, the two programs will work in tandem. The amount received from both programs combined generally may not exceed 80 percent of your pre-disability income. Social Security benefits are considered primary in nature, and the compensation awarded by your private insurer will probably be reduced to meet that 80 percent threshold.

Once a positive decision is rendered, you will continue to have obligations under both Social Security and short-term and long-term disability programs. Under both you should continue to obtain medical treatment for your impairment from a health care provider. Your condition may be one that could improve with continued therapy or new technologies, enabling you to return to the workplace in the future. Even if your situation remains static or deteriorates, documentation is required, as your circumstances will be reviewed on a periodic basis to determine whether benefits continue to be warranted.

While on Social Security disability insurance benefits, you can continue to work as long as your monthly income does not exceed a specified amount determined by the Administration. At present, you may earn up to $725 per month, not including disability benefits. If you make more than this amount, it is considered to be a "trial work period."

If you exceed the income limit nine times in a 60-month period, Social Security will stop your benefits for months when your earnings are considered "substantial," presently that is, if they exceed $860 per month. Further, during the 36-month period following the end of the trial work period, your benefits can be restarted if your earnings fall below the substantial level and your disabling condition persists. In each instance, you are notified of the Administration's decision by letter, explaining their reasoning and offering the opportunity to appeal.

Under a short-term or long-term disability contract, in addition to the obligation to seek medical treatment for the disabling condition on an ongoing basis, you must make sure that the health care provider sends copies of your medical records to the disability insurance company regularly. Failure to provide this information may form the basis for a termination of benefits, even though the disabling condition remains. Treatment must continue, and the records relating to medical examinations must be forwarded to the disability insurance carrier.

Social Security disability insurance benefits continue until either the disabling condition disappears or you reach retirement age under the rules of the Administration. At retirement the payments will continue, but instead of being called disability benefits, they will be considered a retirement distribution and will be subject to the rules governing such income.

Social Security supplemental disability benefits continue until your condition improves, you reach retirement age, or you no longer qualify financially. It is your obligation to notify the Social Security Administration of any changes that would warrant a change of benefits. Future payments, including retirement benefits, could be withheld if you fail to timely inform the Administration of any such change.

Long-term disability is based in contract. The payment of long-term disability will be terminated when the contractual obligation to pay those benefits ceases. Under the insurer's guidelines, this could be a specified number of months following the beginning of benefits, or at age 65, or when retirement distributions are to begin.

The information in this chapter is not intended to be all-inclusive with regard to the various disability benefits available to you. It is, instead, intended to provide a general overview. If you want detailed information on a specific program, I recommend that you contact the Social Security Administration, your employer, and your insurer. Finally, in addition to these sources, should you have questions concerning your rights under any disability program, you should consult with an attorney familiar with this area of law.

Chapter 13
The Personal Cost of Pain

🌾 *Relationships*

Pain affects not only you but also those around you.

PEOPLE EXPERIENCE THE PHYSICAL sensation of pain alone, but the emotional, practical, and interpersonal consequences of pain are experienced by the patient's friends and family as well as by the patient. If the person in pain has a life partner, the pain adds a different dimension to the relationship. For example, the patient may have been a major income contributor in the past but now is unable to contribute financially to the relationship. Formerly, the patient's religious faith may have been unflappable, but in this new reality, he or she may be more questioning—and this questioning may unsettle or upset the partner if the partner has a strong religious faith. Until recently the relationship may have included an active sexual component, but now intimacy may be rare. The life that may have been a joy yesterday may feel like a burden today. For both the patient and his or her partner, it is very important to find satisfaction and fulfillment together.

We all are part of groups. At home we are part of a couple, a family, and an extended family with parents, siblings, and other relatives. We are part of a community—we live around others, shop together, and pray together. Our interpersonal relationships are an important part of our health. One of the worst aspects of pain is that it can cause us to isolate ourselves from the people who complete our lives. People in pain need to work hard to maintain their social connections.

People who remain engaged with the people around them tend to cope better with their pain. Some people feel that talking about their problems is a burden to other people, but this is often not the case, because sharing one's experience with others may be beneficial for everyone. The person with pain has an outlet for his or her concerns, and the person listening has an opportunity to feel needed and provide help.

People who maintain their connections with others are better able to avoid or recover from depression, are able to ease their stress, and live longer. As noted earlier in this book, pain can contribute to clinical depression or feeling blue, but people who stay involved with the people around them are provided with a distraction and are less focused on themselves and their current condition. Although clinical depression is a physiological phenomenon, how it is experienced and its duration can be altered by environment. Pain is a major stressor, and stress ages a person prematurely. Studies show that by actively participating in a social unit, people can ease their tension and even prolong their lives.[1] Positive interaction can also show a patient that he or she is not alone and that others who have chronic conditions can and do live seemingly normal lives.

People with pain need to maintain and even expand their connections with others; they should avoid if at all possible falling prey to self-pity. They should participate in family activities and other social occasions. They should answer telephone calls, respond to letters, and accept invitations to outings. Patients must be receptive and accommodating and expect the same in return. As is true in all relationships, communication is a key ingredient for success.

Adjusting Relationships | How friends and family can help

If someone close to you is suffering from pain, you can help. First learn about pain; find out what others have discovered in their journey to help someone living with pain. Teach yourself not to "enable," not to be at the whim of the person with pain. Rather, help him or her to live a normal life and achieve as much independence as possible. Do not make his or her discomfort the focus of every conversation; there is more to people than the pain they are managing. Make sure that some of your interactions don't even mention the condition.

Being overly attentive to a person in pain may decrease his or her sense of independence and even increase the perception of pain. Give your loved one room to learn to manage circumstances and do not react to every grimace, groan, or sigh. That is, respond to the general circumstance of your loved one living with pain, but do not respond each time the pain is mentioned. Keep him or her involved. Let the individual know that you want to continue to do the things you previously enjoyed together, and that you are willing to accommodate his or her physical needs.

Listen to your loved one. Give positive support when appropriate. Occasional problem solving can be helpful, but encourage him or her be as self-sufficient as possible. Finally, remember to take care of yourself. When a loved one develops a chronic condition, it's easy to become so focused on being the assistant that you neglect your own needs. Allowing your physical, mental, and spiritual state to deteriorate will compromise your ability to be helpful.

Improving Relationships | What the patient can do

If you are personally suffering from pain, you should share your feelings about your challenges with your family and friends. Be mindful, however, that while venting can be helpful, it should never be one-sided. Just as was true before the onset of your condition, it remains important even now: You need to be receptive to the problems of others, as well.

Pain can tempt you to withdraw, but that will ultimately leave you isolated with only your pain as company, and withdrawal frustrates others. Those around you may lose their attachment to you and stop understanding what you are going through. Communicating with close friends and family is essential, but it should be done thoughtfully. For some, letting them know you are having a bad day is sufficient; for others, you may have to provide an extensive explanation. Communicate symptoms but do not vent negative emotions. The glass can be either half empty or half full and viewing it as the latter is definitely more pleasant for both you and your support network. Long-term whining and anger alienate others and will not elicit the understanding you need.

Communication is the key in helping others to understand what you are experiencing. But these channels may get blocked. Especially in close relationships, such as with life partners, it is important to recognize stresses and discuss them with the other person. You may need a counselor's help to get through this together. Another way to improve your communication skills is to record your feelings in a journal. Journaling can help you to understand yourself better, and an improved awareness will help you to communicate with others more effectively.

If your condition keeps you from doing things that you previously enjoyed with others, like taking a daily walk, look for new ways to interact with friends. Letting them know you can still walk, but at a slower pace, tells them you still want their companionship. Find other activities to enjoy together.

Trying to remain positive when discussing your new challenges doesn't mean you can't be honest. Telling friends who ask about you that you are learning to manage chronic low back pain is positive; telling them you are drowning in your pain and don't know how you'll make it to the next day will overwhelm them.

Back pain undoubtedly impairs your ability to function at previous levels. You may find it difficult now to accomplish simple tasks, so pacing is important. You may need to ask others for a helping hand. Friendships can improve with adversity; friends like to be supportive and helpful.

Be receptive to compliments. When people come to understand your pain state and how you are controlling its impact on your life, they will be impressed. They may also learn important coping skills and life perspectives from you. Be gracious in receiving their compliments.

Relationships can be strained or strengthened during challenging times. Believe in yourself and believe in the people you care about and who care about you.

Appendix
The Anatomy of the Back

THE BACK IS MADE up of bones, discs, spinal cord, nerves, ligaments, blood supply, and muscles. Your physician will consider all of these parts of the back in trying to identify the cause of your pain. Follow along with the illustrations in this chapter to get a better sense of the anatomy of the back.

Before beginning, it will be useful to define the terms collagen and fibers. *Collagen* is a protein found in many structures in the body, such as discs (the back's "shock absorbers"), ligaments (which connect bones to each other), and fibrous tissue. It is the primary *protein of connective tissue* and the most common protein in humans. Collagen makes up about 2 percent of muscle tissue and 6 percent of the weight of some of our strongest muscles.

A fiber can be thought of as being like a length of thread; the word *fibers* describes the appearance of a wide range of structures in the body, such as ligaments, tendons, and fascia. When multiple fibers make up a sheet of tissue, this is called a *fibrous sheet*.

You don't have to remember all of the details of this appendix or the technical terms used, but by reading it you may get a better sense of the part of your anatomy that is the source of your pain.

Bones | Starting with our skeleton

The bones in the back are called *vertebrae*. The spine is divided into four regions: the *cervical spine* (the neck), the *thoracic spine* (the middle of the back), the *lumbar spine*, and the *sacrum*. The lumbar and sacral vertebrae combined are considered the low back. The low back has five separated lumbar vertebrae, five fused sacral vertebrae (sacrum), and four partially fused lumbar vertebrae (coccyx). The lumbar spine is where most problems related to low back pain are thought to occur.

The sacrum is located at the base of the spine and joins with the pelvis; back pain related to this structure tends to occur in relation to the joint connecting to the pelvis, known as the sacroiliac joint. The sacrum is important in supporting the lumbar vertebrae and transferring the weight of your trunk to the pelvis and legs. The coccyx tends to be a benign structure unless you fall on it; a painful localized condition called coccydynia can develop when you injure your "tailbone."

The lumbar vertebrae are separated from each other in the front (anterior) by discs and in the back (posterior) by the facets, or zygapophyseal joints. The vertebrae are numbered starting from the head (superior) to the toe (inferior): one through five. The vertebrae have different structures: body, pedicles, lamina, spinous processes, and two superior and inferior articular processes.

The vertebral body is the largest part of the vertebrae; it has a blocklike appearance. It's a very vascular structure, which means that it contains many blood vessels. The term "broken back" usually refers to a fracture of this part of the vertebra, which is considered a compression fracture.

Pedicles project posteriorly from the vertebral body. The area between the pedicles superiorly and inferiorly is where nerve roots pass on their way to forming important nerves for the lower torso and legs. Extending posteriorly from the pedicle are the lamina; these structures angle toward the midline. The articular processes extend from the junction of the lamina and pedicles superiorly and inferiorly respectively; the junction between articular processes is a synovial joint covered with cartilage. Bone that juts laterally from the junction of the pedicle and lamina is called the transverse process. The spinous process is located at the junction of the lamina.

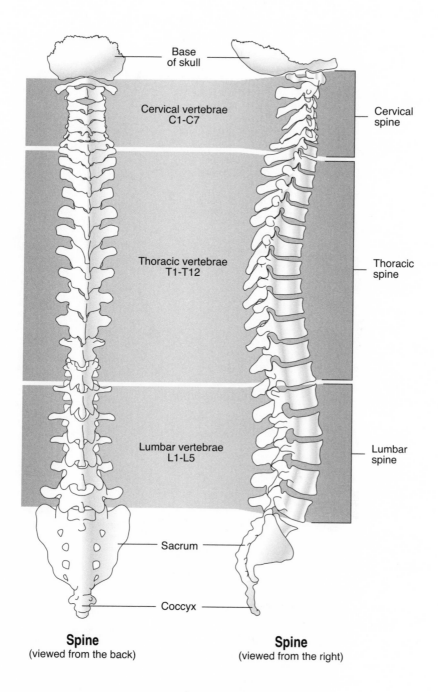

Base
of skull

Cervical vertebrae
C1-C7

Cervical
spine

Thoracic vertebrae
T1-T12

Thoracic
spine

Lumbar vertebrae
L1-L5

Lumbar
spine

Sacrum

Coccyx

Spine
(viewed from the back)

Spine
(viewed from the right)

Back and side views of the spine, including lumbar spine

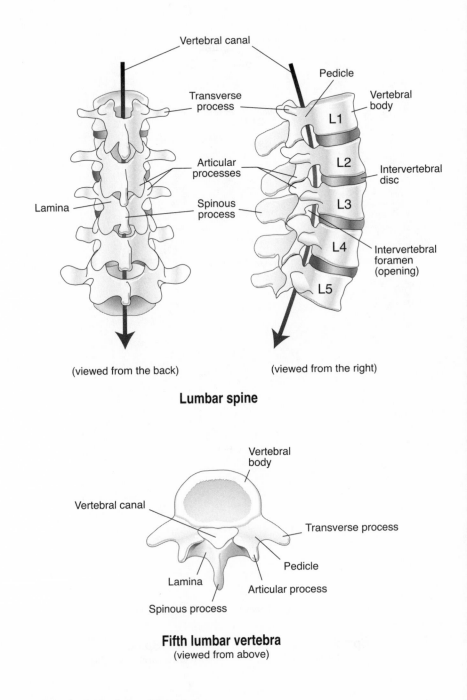

Lumbar spine

Vertebral canal

Transverse process

Articular processes

Lamina

Spinous process

(viewed from the back)

Vertebral canal

Pedicle

Vertebral body

L1

L2

L3

L4

L5

Intervertebral disc

Intervertebral foramen (opening)

(viewed from the right)

Fifth lumbar vertebra
(viewed from above)

Vertebral body

Vertebral canal

Transverse process

Lamina

Pedicle

Articular process

Spinous process

Top: Back and side views of the spine
Bottom: A single lumbar vertebra

Vertebral Canal | The canal that contains our spinal cord

The opening within the vertebrae is called the vertebral foramen; the foramens together compose the vertebral canal. Superiorly the lumbar vertebrae surround the spinal cord. Inferior to the spinal cord are nerve roots that travel to the various intervertebral foramen and form nerves; as a group these nerve roots are called the cauda equina because they resemble "a horse's tail." Nerves leaving the canal in the lumbar region exit via the intervertebral foramens.

Discs | The soft cushions in our back

Intervertebral discs are located between the vertebrae. The shock-absorbing central component of the disc is called the nucleus pulposus. Surrounding the nucleus is the annulus fibrosus. Below and above the nucleus are cartilaginous supporting structures called endplates.

Most of the nucleus pulposus is composed of water. Proteoglycans are molecules that help keep the water in place. As people age, the water content decreases and this tissue loses its elasticity; as a result the height of the disc decreases. In people with disc disease, proteoglycans are replaced with fibrocartilage that binds to less water. These changes in composition, primarily as a result of aging, account for the fact that we shrink in height as we age.

The nucleus pulposus functions like a shock-absorbing sponge completely enclosed in a fibrous container. In a healthy disc, stresses are disbursed easily throughout the disc. In a diseased disc, stresses are disbursed disproportionately in the periphery.

The primary component of the annulus fibrosus is water. Its primary dry component is collagen. (Remember that collagen is a protein commonly found in fibrous tissues.) The fibers that make up the annulus fibrosus are grouped into sheets that crisscross with other fibrous sheets while connecting to the vertebral bodies. Vertically oriented fibers function to resist flexion, extension, and lateral bending motions of the spine. The horizontal collagen fibers resist rotational motions of the spine. These functions help provide stability to the spine.

All structures in the body degenerate over time, and the spine is no exception. Loss of elasticity in our tissues is one of the hallmarks of the

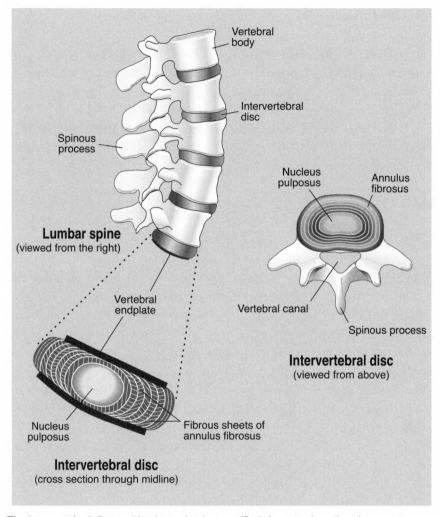

The intervertebral disc and lumbar spine in magnified views to show the placement, structure, and composition of these parts of the back

aging process. It is the loss of tissue elasticity that causes our skin to wrinkle. In the disc, the loss of elasticity of tissue most commonly seen is the part of the disc closest to the nerve as it exits from the spine. Herniations occur when something in the body protrudes into another part of the body where it should not be. In a herniated disc, the nucleus pulposus of the disc protrudes through a degenerated annulus fibrosus.

The disc receives nutrition primarily through the vertebral endplate. Nutrients pass through the endplate to reach the rest of the disc. When

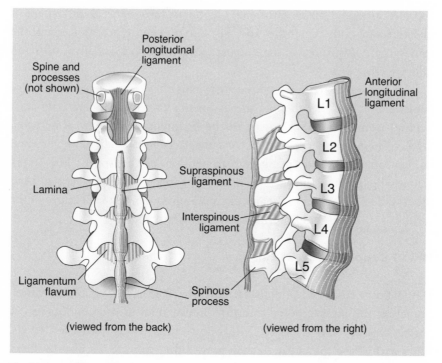

Posterior
longitudinal
ligament

Spine and
processes
(not shown)

Anterior
longitudinal
ligament

L1

L2

Supraspinous
ligament

Lamina

L3

Interspinous
ligament

L4

Ligamentum
flavum

L5

Spinous
process

(viewed from the back)   (viewed from the right)

The lumbar spine and its ligaments

the endplate becomes calcified—again, generally as a result of aging—nutrient transport to the disc can be impaired, potentially leading to overall decreased health of the disc.

Many people have doubted that a disc could be a source of pain, but recent studies have supported the idea that it can be.[1] A relatively new finding is that in healthy discs, nerve fiber endings can be found in the periphery of the annulus fibrosus. Studies have also shown that with aging and other changes in the disc, the nerve fibers will grow even farther into the disc. Now that we know that the disc is a potential source of pain, therapy can be directed to alleviating pain caused by the discs.

Spinal Ligaments | Holding our bones together

Ligaments are elastic, fibrous tissues that connect bones to each another. The two primary spinal ligaments are the anterior and posterior longitudinal ligaments, which connect one vertebral body to another both in front and in back of the vertebral body. Ligaments also attach to the superior and inferior endplates of vertebrae. Ligaments resist vertical movement of one vertebral body to another and they also prevent hyperextension of the spine. Again, a purpose of these structures is to provide stability and avoid injury to the spine.

The ligamenta flava are paired ligaments that connect one lamina to another. Some of the fibers of the ligamenta flava (which primarily connect adjacent lamina) also assist in the ligamental connections between facets. These ligaments resist excess displacement of adjacent vertebral lamina, therefore preventing hyperextension of the spine. The interspinous ligament connects one spinous process to the adjacent spinous process. The supraspinous ligament runs behind the posterior edges of the spinous processes, bridging the interspinous spaces.

Blood Supply | Going with the flow

Blood flows from the abdominal aorta to the vertebrae. Blood vessels branch at the intervertebral foramina and extend to surrounding structures. Typically blood vessels will follow the pathway of nerves. In the bony part of the spinal canal, they pass to the endplate. In healthy discs, no blood vessels exist. Blood returns to the heart through veins. Veins in the spine follow the path of the arteries that supply it.

Back Muscles | Making it work

Muscles originate and insert into the bones in the lumbar spine and the neighboring structures. Many groups of muscles work together or in opposition to each other. Their orientation allows flexion, extension, lateral flexion, and rotation of the spine. The extensor muscles run parallel to the spine and extend and laterally flex the spine. The abdominal muscles flex back and forth and rotate the spine.

Spinal Cord | Our inner core

The spinal cord extends from the brain stem at the base of the skull to the upper lumbar vertebrae (L1 or L2). Extending from the distal end of the cord (the end farthest from the brain) are rootlets that resemble a horse's tail, known as the cauda equina. Nerve rootlets extend from the spinal

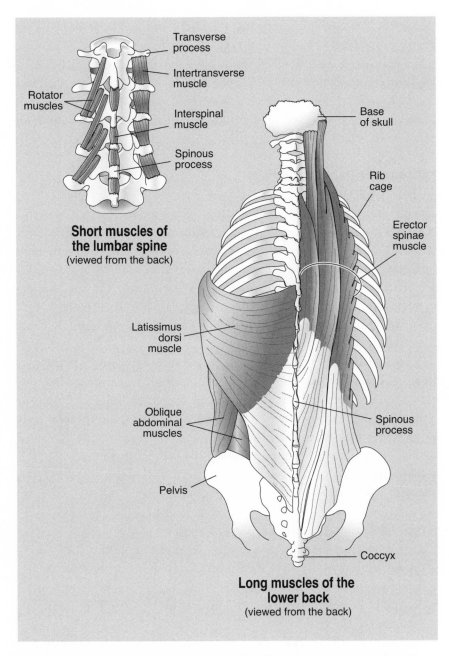

Short muscles of the lumbar spine
(viewed from the back)

Transverse process

Intertransverse muscle

Rotator muscles

Interspinal muscle

Spinous process

Base of skull

Rib cage

Erector spinae muscle

Latissimus dorsi muscle

Oblique abdominal muscles

Spinous process

Pelvis

Coccyx

Long muscles of the lower back
(viewed from the back)

The back muscles. Back view of the spine, showing ribs, erector spinae muscle, and deeper intervertebral muscles cord to the nerve opening at nearly every level of the spinal column; root-lets from one level can join rootlets from another level and form nerves.

A nerve from each level of the lumbar vertebrae has branches to all neighboring structures: the spinal column—including the facet, the blood vessels, muscle, and skin. The spine is covered in a sack of tissue called the meninges; the spinal fluid flows inside the meninges and surrounds the spinal cord.

Anatomy of Pain | Why it hurts

Changes in normal anatomic structures can cause disease that manifests as pain. But even when an anatomic alteration is found, it is not necessarily the cause of low back pain. Nevertheless, doctors tend to assume that a patient's sensation of low back pain arises from altered anatomy, and that the altered anatomy explains why the back hurts. On the contrary, however, the altered anatomy may not explain the back pain. For the most part, low back pain is nonspecific; it can occur from normal or from abnormal structures.

A vocabulary of terms is used to describe various processes in the back. Some of these processes are part of the normal course of change during aging, or degeneration, and therefore are not pathologic. Others are pathologic, or are caused by a traumatic event. The spine specialist must use the information provided by the patient and the referring physician to identify which process is responsible for the patient's back pain.

Here are some of the many terms used to describe these processes (many of which are discussed in this book):

- *Spondylosis* is degeneration in the lower back
- *Degenerative disc disease* is the label for degeneration in the discs
- *Spondylolisthesis* is the term used to indicate when one vertebra is displaced in relation to another
- *Stenosis* indicates a narrowing or constriction in a space between vertebrae in the spine
- *Arthropathy* is the term for disease in a joint
- *Fracture* means that bones that should be whole have separated into two or more parts
- *Strains* or *sprains* refer to tears in ligaments, tendons, or supporting soft tissue structures

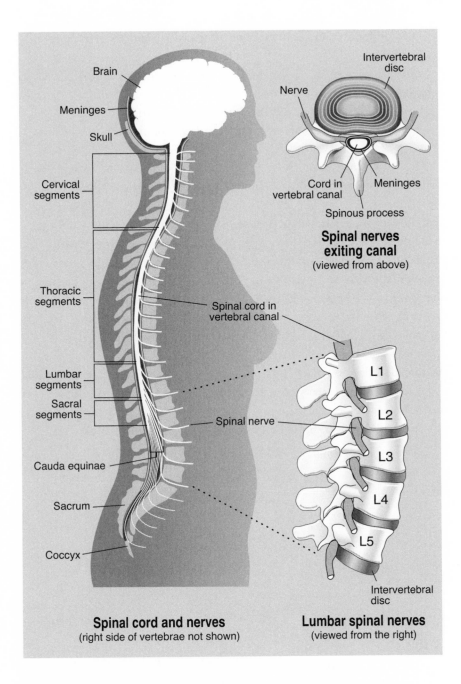

Spinal nerves exiting canal
(viewed from above)

Spinal cord and nerves
(right side of vertebrae not shown)

Lumbar spinal nerves
(viewed from the right)

The central nervous system. A cross-sectional view of the spine and lower skull, showing the meninges, brain, spinal cord, cauda equina, and spinal nerves

- *Kyphosis* denotes an abnormal posterior protrusion (back to front) of the spine
- *Scoliosis* indicates an irregular lateral (side-to-side) curvature of the spine.
- *Paget's disease* refers to an unhealthy excess growth of bone
- *Osteoporosis* means a state of bone with low calcification

Back problems can also develop as a result of cancer. Infection can occur in the bone, the disc, or in the space between the spinal cord and the bone. Structures not located in the back can also cause pain that is perceived in the back. Pelvic organs, such as the prostate, and endometrial tissue or pelvic infections may be sensed in the back. Kidney disease, like stones and infection, though usually perceived in the flanks (your sides, between the ribs and pelvis), may be perceived in the back. Pathologic alteration of the abdominal aorta, such as an aneurysm, may be sensed in the back. Finally, disease in various gastrointestinal structures, like the pancreas, gall bladder, and bowel may translate into back pain.

Admittedly, this is a brief anatomy lesson on the back, and there is much more that can be learned from a medical textbook. What is clear even from this short description, however, is that there are plenty of places where a malfunction can occur, and many causes for low back pain.

Notes

Preface

1. Sources differ on the extent of back pain suffered by Americans. See Nisha J. Manek and A. J. MacGregor, "Epidemiology of Back Disorders: Prevalence, Risk Factors, and Prognosis," *Curr Opin Rheumatol* 17, no. 2 (2005): 134–40, ©2005 Lippincott Williams & Wilkins (who give the figure as 61%) and Everett C. Hills, "Mechanical Low Back Pain," Nov. 19, 2009, http://emedicine.medscape.com/article/310353 -overview (who gives the figure as 85%).

Chapter 1. All about Pain

1. Everett C. Hills, "Mechanical Low Back Pain," Nov. 19, 2009, http://emedicine .medscape.com/article/310353-overview.
2. Anthony H. Wheeler, "Pathophysiology of Chronic Back Pain," June 30, 2009, http://emedicine.medscape.com/article/1144130-overview.

Chapter 3. Diagnosing What's Causing Your Pain

1. See http://nccam.nih.gov/health/supplements/wiseuse.htm.

Chapter 5. Exercise for Treating Pain

1. J. Rainville et al., "Exercise as a Treatment for Chronic Low Back Pain," *Spine Journal* 4 (2004): 106–15.

2. L. J. Goodyear, "The Exercise Pill—Too Good to Be True?" *New England Journal of Medicine* 359, no. 17 (2008): 1842–44.

3. See *ACSM's Guidelines for Exercise Testing and Prescription,* 7th Edition (Philadelphia, Lippincott Williams and Wilkins, 2006) and the United States Department of Health and Human Services Web site, www.health.gov/PAGuidelines.

4. See http://www.nhhealthinfo.org/pdf/DHHS-stair-prompts.pdf.

5. J. Rainville and E. P. Frates, "Exercise Tops Options for Back Pain," *Biomechanics* 10, no. 7 (2003): 67–76.

Chapter 6. Tools for Reducing Stress

1. See http://cochrane.org/reviews/en/subtopics/80.html and http://cochrane.org/reviews/en/ab003786.html.

Chapter 7. Pain Medications

1. See A. M. Moultry and I. O. Poon, "The Use of Antidepressants for Chronic Pain," at http://medscape.com/viewarticle/704975.

Chapter 10. Alternative Treatments

1. For more on acupuncture, see the Web site of the National Center for Complementary and Alternative Medicine at http://nccam.nih.gov/health/acupuncture/.

2. A. M. McCaffrey, D. M. Eisenberg, A.T.R. Legedza, R. B. Davis, and R. S. Phillips, "Prayer for Health Concerns: Results of a National Survey on Prevalence and Patterns of Use," *Archives of Internal Medicine* 164 (2004): 858–62. See http://archinte.ama-assn.org/cgi/content/full/164/8/858?SEARCHID=1084721917699_899&hits=10&gca=archinte%3B164%2F8%2F858&FIRSTINDEX=0&FULLTEXT=Anne+M.+McCaffrey&.

Chapter 13. The Personal Cost of Pain

1. Numerous reports link social activity with a reduction in stress. See a summary of B. Farahmand, G. Broman, U. De Faire, D. Vågerö, and A. Ahlbom, "Golf—a Game of Life and Death: Reduced Mortality in Swedish Golf Players," *Scandinavian Journal of Medicine & Science in Sports,* May 30, 2008, found at http://medicalnewstoday.com/articles/109431.php. Stress reduction has also been found to prolong life; see K. Orth-Gomér, N. Schneiderman, H.-X. Wang, C. Walldin, M. Blom, and T.

Jernberg, "Stress Reduction Prolongs Life in Women with Coronary Disease," a study conducted by the Stockholm Women's Intervention Trial for Coronary Heart Disease (SWITCHD) (found at http://circoutcomes.ahajournals.org/cgi/content/full/2/1/25. A summary of the importance of emotional and social support can be found at http://www.stress.org/topic-emotional.htm.

Appendix

1. K. Malik and N. J. Joseph, "Intervertebral Disc a Source of Pain? Low Back Pain: Problems and Future Directions," *Middle East Journal of Anesthesiology* 19, no. 3 (2007): 683–92. See http://www.ncbi.nlm.nih.gov/pubmed/18044296.

Index